Please return or renew this item 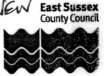 by the last date shown. You may return items to any East Sussex Library. You may renew books by telephone or the internet.

0345 60 80 195 for renewals
0345 60 80 196 for enquiries

**Library and Information Services
eastsussex.gov.uk/libraries**

D0234545

Overcoming Common Problems Series

Selected titles

A full list of titles is available from Sheldon Press,
36 Causton Street, London SW1P 4ST and on our website at
www.sheldonpress.co.uk

The Assertiveness Handbook
Mary Hartley

Breaking Free
Carolyn Ainscough and Kay Toon

Cataract: What You Need to Know
Mark Watts

Cider Vinegar
Margaret Hills

Coping Successfully with Period Problems
Mary-Claire Mason

Coping Successfully with Ulcerative Colitis
Peter Cartwright

Coping Successfully with Your Irritable Bowel
Rosemary Nicol

Coping with Anxiety and Depression
Shirley Trickett

Coping with Blushing
Professor Robert Edelmann

Coping with Bowel Cancer
Dr Tom Smith

Coping with Brain Injury
Maggie Rich

Coping with Chemotherapy
Dr Terry Priestman

Coping with Dyspraxia
Jill Eckersley

Coping with Gout
Christine Craggs-Hinton

Coping with Heartburn and Reflux
Dr Tom Smith

Coping with Macular Degeneration
Dr Patricia Gilbert

Coping with Polycystic Ovary Syndrome
Christine Craggs-Hinton

Coping with Postnatal Depression
Sandra L. Wheatley

Coping with a Stressed Nervous System
Dr Kenneth Hambly and Alice Muir

Depressive Illness
Dr Tim Cantopher

Eating Disorders and Body Image
Christine Craggs-Hinton

Free Your Life from Fear
Jenny Hare

Help Your Child Get Fit Not Fat
Jan Hurst and Sue Hubberstey

Helping Children Cope with Anxiety
Jill Eckersley

How to Beat Pain
Christine Craggs-Hinton

How to Cope with Difficult People
Alan Houel and Christian Godefroy

How to Keep Cholesterol in Check
Dr Robert Povey

Living with Asperger Syndrome
Dr Joan Gomez

Living with Autism
Fiona Marshall

Living with Fibromyalgia
Christine Craggs-Hinton

Living with Food Intolerance
Alex Gazzola

Living with Loss and Grief
Julia Tugendhat

Living with Lupus
Philippa Pigache

Living with Rheumatoid Arthritis
Philippa Pigache

Living with Sjögren's Syndrome
Sue Dyson

Losing a Child
Linda Hurcombe

Making Relationships Work
Alison Waines

Overcoming Loneliness and Making Friends
Márianna Csóti

Treating Arthritis – The Drug-Free Way
Margaret Hills

Understanding Obsessions and Compulsions
Dr Frank Tallis

Overcoming Common Problems

Living with Osteoporosis

Second edition

Joan Gomez

sheldon **PRESS**

First published in Great Britain in 2000

Sheldon Press
36 Causton Street
London SW1P 4ST

Second edition published 2006

Copyright © Dr Joan Gomez 2000, 2006

All rights reserved. No part of this book may be reproduced
or transmitted in any form or by any means, electronic or
mechanical, including photocopying, recording, or by any
information storage and retrieval system, without permission
in writing from the publisher.

The author and publisher have made every effort to
ensure that external website and email addresses are
correct and up to date at the time of going to press. The
author and publisher are not responsible for the content,
quality or continuing accessibility of the sites.

British Library Cataloguing-in-Publication Data

A catalogue record for this book is available
from the British Library

ISBN-13: 978–0–85969–960–0
ISBN-10: 0–85969–960–9

Typeset by Deltatype Limited, Birkenhead, Merseyside
Printed in Great Britain by
Ashford Colour Press

Contents

Introduction: What osteoporosis is and
why it is important to you   1

1 Your living bones   3
2 How osteoporosis shows itself   8
3 Types of osteoporosis   19
4 Secondary osteoporosis   28
5 The risks   35
6 Finding out: Diagnostic tests   42
7 Treatment 1: Hormonal   50
8 Treatment 2: Calcium   62
9 Treatment 3: Bisphosphonates and recent
   advances – teriparatide   67
10 Getting over a broken hip and other fractures   75
11 Falls   88
12 Moods and emotions   93
13 Prevention 1: Lifestyle and exercise   98
14 Prevention 2: Nourishing your bones   105

   Useful addresses   115
   Index   119

Introduction: What osteoporosis is and why it is important to you

You are in danger of osteoporosis – maybe not immediately, but certainly by the time you hit 40, or if you are unlucky, years before that. It is not something you can laugh off – it can mean long-term pain, crippling deformity from broken and crumbling bones and a 20 per cent chance of premature death. And it does not only happen to other people. It has reached epidemic proportions in North America and Western Europe.

In the UK you run a lifetime risk of one in three if you are a woman or one in twelve for a man. The odds shorten to one in two and one in eight, respectively, from age 60 onwards. By that time there is a 25 per cent likelihood of having a crush fracture in one or more vertebrae (the small bones that make up the spinal column), and a staggering 30 per cent risk of hip fracture. The American figures are no better, particularly for white women and other Caucasians – the light-skinned races. It is estimated that more than 50 per cent of them already show evidence of osteoporosis by the time they are 45, jumping to 85 per cent for the over-seventies. It is the commonest chronic disease among American women.

Put another way, the risk of sustaining a broken hip due to osteoporosis is greater than that of cancer of the breast, ovaries and uterus added to-gether – with a 20 per cent likelihood of dying within the year. The health bill for problems related to osteoporosis is astronomical and the costs are escalating all the time. While the individual costs per patient are in fact decreasing, there is an annual increase of 10 per cent in the number of people with the condition. Because we are all living longer nowadays, there is a steadily increasing number of over-sixties, the group most vulnerable to osteoporosis. Osteologists – bone experts – calculate that there will be six-and-a-quarter million hip fractures worldwide in the year 2050. Currently, in the UK alone, more than a thousand people a week suffer a hip fracture due to osteoporosis.

What is this disorder that can wreak such havoc?

The word osteoporosis, from the Greek for 'bone' and 'pore', tells us that the affected bones have holes in their structure. Although the bones are the same size as normal externally, except for the vertebrae which are crushed, there is less actual bone material in their composition. This makes them fragile and easily broken – like Aero chocolate compared with a solid bar.

Why does this happen and what is the link with getting older?

It is one of nature's neat arrangements that can misfire. Up to the age of 35 to 40 we are likely to need good strong bones and muscles, for possible manual work if we are male, and carrying and coping with children if we are female. From around then onwards the physical demands on our bodies lessen. You will not be toting a heavy toddler around when you are 50 or playing football for cash. Since it is no longer necessary to have such a substantial skeleton to lug around, your bones fine down and get lighter, while your muscles, to match, lose some of their power. The trouble is that the process can overrun and your bones may become dangerously breakable. This is osteoporosis.

While it affects older people most commonly, do not fool yourself that there is no danger when you are younger. There is a juvenile form which affects children; in some cases it follows childbirth in a 20- or 30-year-old; and it frequently results from taking steroid medication at any age. Several chronic illnesses, for example rheumatoid arthritis, multiple sclerosis and anorexia, and even persistent dieting can lead to osteoporosis sooner or later.

Some risk is unavoidable in your later years, but the outlook is not all doom and gloom.

Osteoporosis is preventable

The precautions you need to take are cheap and simple. The only proviso is that you start them as soon as possible. Ideally your mother will have set you on the right path in your first two decades, but more likely it will be when you are an adult in your own right that you may start to think of adopting a safety-first lifestyle – in relation to osteoporosis.

Most likely of all it will not be until you are 50-plus, taking stock of your first half-century, that you will seriously consider protecting yourself against this damaging condition. It is still not too late, but increasingly urgent, to take evasive action. If you were heading for a collision in your car would you try swerving and slamming on the brakes right up to the moment of impact? The principle is exactly the same. Prevention is immensely worthwhile.

Nor is there any need for despair if you have already suffered from an osteoporotic fracture – the late Queen Mother, for example, recovered marvellously well from a broken hip at 98. There is plenty that you can do, still, to combat osteoporosis, but whatever your age and situation – start now.

1

Your living bones

Do you think of bones as dull, dry-as-dust and inert, of interest only to your dog? Nothing could be farther from the truth. Your bones, at this moment, are active, vital bodily organs constantly changing and reforming, and intimately involved with your metabolism: the way the body works chemically.

The most notable characteristic of bone is its rigidity. If it was as flexible as other tissues you would be a shapeless mass, like a bin-liner full of rubbish, but in a bag of skin instead of plastic. On the other hand, if your bones were solid right through, they would be too heavy to manage. The secret of bone is in its structure, which is unlike any other tissue. Each bone comprises the cortex and the trabecular part. *Cortex* is the Latin for 'bark', and it refers to the hard, compact casing of the bone. It accounts for 80 per cent of the total bone material. The trabecular part, from the Latin *trabeculum*, or 'beam', is a scaffolding supporting the cortex, making up the remaining 20 per cent of bone tissue, but occupying more space, comparatively.

The matrix or background tissue consists mainly of the protein collagen, and also contains the bone cells or osteocytes. They control the metabolism of the living, changing bone, including its mineral content. This is largely calcium phosphate, which gives the bone its strength, but it also includes some sodium, magnesium and fluoride.

The osteocytes

These comprise two main types.

- *Osteoclasts* – Greek for 'bone-breakers'. They are in charge of the demolition work, the destruction and removal of outdated bone tissue.
- *Osteoblasts* – named from the Greek for 'germs', meaning origins, as in the germ of an idea. They put in train the process of building new, replacement tissue. They alter in shape when they reach the stage of laying down calcium in the immature bone, and again, finally, when they enter a resting phase.

Your bones, like the rest of your body, are in a constant state of flux, discarding old tissue and replacing it with fresh, new material. Your red blood cells are renewed every six weeks, and you can see for yourself your new nail tissue growing all the time. During childhood the whole of the skeleton is replaced, cell by cell, every two years; as an adult this takes

3

seven to ten years. This constant renewal is the essence of life, and allows for the repair of injuries and a certain degree of recovery from the ageing process. With bone this process, which includes remodelling, is particularly important during periods of growth. If their bones just became bigger all over children could never grow taller.

The bone cycle

- *Activation* is the first event. Gangs of osteoclasts are attracted to sites on the inner surfaces of the bones. This happens at regular intervals in the ordinary way, but may be stimulated by, for example, an injury, or, paradoxically, too long a rest.
- *Resorption* is the process of breaking down the selected, tiny areas of bone to form little pits. It is carried out by the osteoclasts and takes four to twelve days.
- *Reversal* consists of filling in the little hollows left by the osteoclasts with a temporary cement. The cells responsible are called reversal cells and their work takes seven to ten days.
- *Coupling* takes place when resorption and reversal are complete. It is triggered by the reversal cells when they have completed their task, sending out a 'come-hither' signal to the osteoblasts. These now take over.
- *Formation* is the main bone rebuilding or re-forming process, starting with the production of layers of matrix.
- *Mineralization*, the final stage, is the laying down of calcium and the other minerals in the new bone.

The removal and replacement of old tissues normally involves only 10 per cent of the bone at any one time, and goes on simultaneously in different sites, with four times as much activity in the trabecular bone as in the cortical parts. This is because it has much more surface area to work on, with its cross bars and strands. While resorption takes only a matter of days, the building up and mineralizing aspects of the cycle take months. This means that unless the turnover runs to a very slow timescale, the resorption side gets ahead of the rebuilding, and the net result is a loss of bone. Chemical clues that resorption is actively proceeding are the presence of hydroxyproline in your water and alkaline phosphatase in your blood.

The balance

During your childhood, especially the first two to three years, and again during your pubertal growth spurt, much more building than breaking down takes place. This bias diminishes gradually during early adulthood and in the period from around 25 to 35 the two processes are in balance: you neither gain nor lose bone.

Thirty-five, give or take a year or so, is a watershed in the dynamic life of your bones. Now the balance tips decisively to the side of resorption. We all gradually lose bony tissue and with it the mineral, or calcium, content. The parts most affected are the trabecular areas. The 'scaffolding' becomes lighter and more sparse – and weaker – and every cycle now means a further loss. Osteoporosis is setting in.

Unfortunately, you will not be aware of all this happening. Not for nothing is osteoporosis called 'the silent calcium thief'. You are unlikely to have any recognizable symptoms until you have had the disorder for several years, and X-rays will not show the loss of bone tissue until it has reached at least 40 per cent. By that time your bones are already in the danger bracket for breaking or being crushed out of shape with little or no apparent cause. Such events are frequently the first indication of anything being amiss; they are most likely to occur when you are over 60.

Each cycle of bone activity leaves a deficit and this is greatly increased when there is an increase in the rate of bone turnover. This occurs in several situations. The most important of these is the menopause, the mid-life upheaval in female hormones. Other hormonal changes, certain medicines, bodily inactivity – for instance during a physical illness and convalescence – and ageing itself, all accelerate bone metabolism and lead to osteoporosis.

Injury acts similarly, including *tissue fatigue*: this is due to a summation of the constant small physical stresses of living. It is analogous to metal fatigue in engineering, and affects only rigid structures, in this case the bones. There is an obvious short-term benefit in bone resorption and renewal for the repair of injury of any type, but the price is an increase in long-term bone loss. If you break a bone in an accident when you are 40-plus, however well it heals there is an overall loss of bone tissue.

Peak bone mass

This means the sum total of your bony tissue when it reached its maximum in your early twenties. Although your bones stop growing in length at the age of 16–18, they continue to increase in density and strength for several more years. Calcium is already being laid down in the unborn baby's bones during the last three months of pregnancy. At birth the infant has about 25 mg of calcium in his bones and this increases to around 1000 mg in maturity.

Men have larger bones and so a greater initial mass of bone substance than women, while black people of both sexes have considerably more than whites. Bone mass is important for the future, like money in the bank. If you have a sizeable reserve to start with, the small regular withdrawals that come later will not lead to bankruptcy, or in the case of your bones, osteoporosis. This is a good reason to take care that youngsters from birth to the age of 21 have plenty of nourishment, including sufficient calcium and vitamin D.

Other factors affecting peak bone mass include family history. If your mother or other relatives have been osteoporosis victims, you are at extra risk. It is bad news, too, if you have been prevented from taking regular exercise because of some physical handicap or illness – fortunately poliomyelitis is no longer a factor. Smoking, excessive alcohol intake and delayed puberty (sometimes due to athletic training or anorexia nervosa), and another hormonal disorder, premenstrual tension, also militate against building up a substantial peak bone mass. Space travel does the same, but does not affect many of us, while there is uncertainty about the effects of the contraceptive pill, having a baby and breastfeeding.

What your bones need to lead their active life

The two basic requirements are food and exercise.

Food

What you eat has a major effect on the health and strength of your bones and your chances of avoiding or reducing the risk of osteoporosis – or worsening it. Calcium is vital for bone-building and dairy products, such as milk, cheese and yoghurt, are particularly rich in this mineral. However, they may not provide the most efficient way of absorbing it. Babies, for instance, obtain more calcium from their mothers' watery milk than from cows' milk, which contains four times as much.

Protein is an essential building block but, due to its acidity, leaches out calcium from the bones and teeth. Red meat is particularly potent in this respect and Cheddar cheese even more so. A hard cheese diet leaves your body with less rather than more calcium in its bone store. Soft, fizzy drinks contain high levels of phosphorus, which also draws on the calcium reserve to neutralize it. Caffeine, in coffee, tea and chocolate, also salt, sugar and alcohol, result in extra calcium being lost in the urine. In addition alcohol diminishes the activity of the bone-building osteoblasts and reduces calcium absorption in the intestines. Tannin in tea together with iron also blocks the absorption of calcium. Bran, often taken for its laxative effect or as a breakfast dish, contains phytates. These bind and excrete such valuable minerals as zinc and magnesium – and calcium. Green vegetables such as broccoli are basically alkaline and counteract the acid foods, but rhubarb and spinach, although alkaline, react with calcium, preventing its absorption.

Increasing age is accompanied by a loss of the ability to deal with acids and an increased vulnerability to degenerative diseases such as arthritis or cancer.

Diet will often supply all the calcium you need, but supplements are readily available in tablet form. Extra calcium is beneficial for most of the elderly, and mandatory for anyone who has recently suffered a fracture because of osteoporosis. It is never too late to start taking calcium. The appropriate quantities are discussed in detail in Chapter 8.

In relation to calcium, vitamin D (cholecalciferol) is like the ignition key of your car – calcium is unusable without it. Calcium deficiency is often secondary to a lack of vitamin D.

Vitamin D is called the 'sunshine' vitamin because we humans can manufacture it in our skin when we are exposed to ultraviolet rays. Normally it is enough to go out of doors casually two or three times a week, and we do not need vitamin D from our food. Fatty fish and especially fish liver oils are the best sources if we need to supplement what we can make. Those who may need supplements are the elderly, in temperate climates, especially if they are living in institutions and seldom go outside. A low level of vitamin D cuts down the absorption of calcium from the usual 60 to 80 per cent of what is available to a mere 15 per cent.

Exercise

Weight-bearing exercise is the second requirement for a healthy skeleton. This is the reason for making people stand up on the day after a hip operation, or walk about in a plaster cast when they have broken a leg. If there is no stress on the bones they react by going into resorption and the cycle results in a loss of bone tissue with a danger of osteoporosis. Daily exercise is ideal, but a 40-minute brisk walk three or four times a week is the healthy minimum. Jogging, skipping and impact sports when you are younger are a wonderful insurance against bone rot. See Chapter 13 for an in-depth discussion of lifestyle issues.

What happens if you short-change your bones?

The three possibilities are:
1 *Osteopenia*: all the bones become generally more translucent in an X-ray because there is less solid material, including calcium, in them. Malnutrition and a lack of calcium can cause this condition, which is often a forerunner of osteoporosis.
2 *Rickets and its adult form, osteomalacia*: these comprise a softening of the bones due to a lack of calcium, in turn due to a lack of vitamin D. The result in children is bone deformity and in adults the main symptom is bone pain.
3 *Osteoporosis*: this is a matter not of abnormal bone, but of a shortage of normal bone tissue, due to loss outstripping new bone formation. Poor nourishment and a lack of calcium and vitamin D may contribute to an impairment of bone-tissue manufacture. The bones that result are fragile and brittle.

Always remember your bones are alive – and treat them that way.

2

How osteoporosis shows itself

Osteoporosis sneaks the mineral strength out of your bones without your even knowing, leaving big holes in the honeycomb structure of the inner, trabecular parts. It is like replacing a close-weave fabric with lace – in three dimensions. Your bones become weak and brittle, and liable to break at the slightest jarring, when you are not even aware.

All the symptoms of osteoporosis come from breakages – of two kinds. On the one hand there is the crushing, crumbling, collapsing type of damage to the vertebrae, the column of small bones comprising the spine, while on the other there is what we usually understand by a fracture – a crack or frank break such as can happen to a piece of china. This is the sort that affects the bones which are not part of the backbone, for instance the limb bones, including, most importantly, the hip.

If you have a Ming vase, beautiful but fragile, it will remain intact unless it is subjected to some trauma – a drop or fall, pressure, or repeated minute stresses. It is the same in the case of delicate, osteoporotic bones. The injury that causes it may be so slight that the break seems to be spontaneous. This applies particularly to the vertebrae, but can also occur with a hip fracture. Most people who suffer a broken hip have tripped or slipped from a standing, or sometimes a sitting, position, but there are occasional cases in which it appears that the bone broke first, perhaps from tissue fatigue (see p. 5), and this in turn led to the fall.

Astrid

Astrid was 75, no age these days, and she prided herself on her good health. However, she had been brought up in Norway, where there is very little strong sunshine to enable the skin to make vitamin D. Added to that she was sensitive to lactose (milk sugar), so she had always avoided dairy products, the main source of calcium for most of us. The trouble started, as far as she was aware, when she had a nasty bout of flu which laid her up for nearly three weeks. It was when she started getting up and pottering about that her hip went. She had lost weight and muscle strength during the illness, so the joint had less support than normally – and unbeknown to her, her bones had already been considerably weakened by osteoporosis over a number of years.

All she did was to step off the kerb rather abruptly – and found herself on the ground, in great pain and unable to get up. X-rays in casualty at the local hospital showed a break in the neck of her femur, the angled piece at the upper end of the thigh bone, near the hip joint. The pieces of bone were not out of place, so it was decided to mend Astrid's hip with steel pins. Her GP would have preferred her to have a hip replacement straight off, since this is less liable to post-operative complications than pinning. However, the pinning is a lesser procedure, and the surgeon wanted to avoid Astrid's spending any more time immobilized than necessary. She recovered well, and was walking – and driving – in two months.

Since Astrid was at special risk of another fracture, especially on the other side, she tried wearing a hip protector consisting of foam-padded pants with an outer shell of plastic, intended to reduce the impact of a fall. That was four years ago, but after a few months she gave it up, as did 70 per cent of others who, like her, were over 70 and lived at home. This was partly because of discomfort but more importantly, while there had been a reduction in hip fractures among younger people living in sheltered accommodation or residential care, there was no reduction among the older group, living at home. One study in America found that 90 per cent of patients wearing all-foam pants with no hard plastic were still using them a year later. The nursing staff may have encouraged them. Different types of protector continue to be introduced.

When the substance of the bones is reduced and weakened by osteoporosis, although they keep their size and shape, they are at a high risk of breaking with the smallest injury. The measure that is used to assess this weakness is called bone mineral density (BMD) (see p. 45). A low BMD means a fragile bone and those that may be affected include the limb bones, the hip, pelvis, backbone, collar bone, ribs, hands and feet. The elbow, face and fingers are less susceptible and usually escape the effects of osteoporosis, but that leaves most of the bones in the firing line. The vertebrae, hip and wrist are most commonly affected.

Age itself is a definite factor in liability to fractures of the vertebrae, hip, upper arm, and pelvis in particular, while independently of age and a low BMD, a previous fracture increases the likelihood of another one.

Although the vast majority of hip, wrist and vertebral breaks are due to osteoporosis, there are other possible causes.

- Severe trauma, as in a traffic accident, can break the strongest bone.
- Children and adolescents have weaker bones than adults because they are growing so fast. A two-year-old may easily break an arm falling out of a cot.
- Disorders of bone metabolism make it vulnerable: for example, an excess of parathyroid hormone, the vitamin D deficiency diseases

osteomalacia and rickets, and osteogenesis imperfecta, a developmental disorder.

Fracture of the vertebrae

This is the commonest yet the most deceptive type of fracture. You may be going about for years with a bone in your back slowly crumbling, but be totally unaware. Backache is so common that you are likely to ignore the odd, mild twinge. While osteoporosis has usually made some secret inroads into your bones by the time you are 45 if you are a woman, by 60 the average bone loss amounts to 20 per cent, and there is a one in four – 25 per cent – chance that you have one or more damaged vertebrae. At 65, this has increased to 40 per cent, and by age 75, in 50 per cent of us X-rays will reveal compression fractures in some of our vertebrae. By this age both sexes are vulnerable.

The most obvious indication of vertebral fracture is loss of height. You discover one day that you cannot reach a shelf or window catch which was no problem previously. You must have noticed people talking about 'little old ladies' – but whoever heard anyone mention a 'big old lady'? The discs of gristle between the vertebrae become thinner as you get older and this accounts for some of the apparent shrinkage, but the main loss is due to the slow collapse of the bones themselves – from osteoporosis.

The vertebral bones start off roughly cubical, but as they become more fragile with sparser trabecular scaffolding, the weight of the body and such activities as bending and lifting squash the weakened bone out of shape.

Types of vertebral fracture

1 Crush fracture: the whole bone is compressed and loses height.
2 Endplate type: the top casing of the bone gives way to pressure, making a dip.
3 Anterior wedge fracture: the front of the bone collapses. Ordinary bending movements for picking things up or tying your shoelaces are enough to cause this.

Vertebral fractures arise in two ways. In an *incident* fracture the bone gives way suddenly, perhaps following a trivial injury such as coughing, bending, lifting, sitting down in or getting up from a low chair. A *prevalence* fracture, by contrast, develops gradually, with no definite starting point, but it can result from the same causes in osteoporosis, age-related general deterioration, or, least often, from secondary cancer.

Kirsty

Kirsty's niece was a fast driver. When she took her aunt, for a treat, to a Burns Night concert she pulled up with a flourish outside the Hall, and the older woman was jerked forwards against the pull of her seat belt. She let out a cry. Kirsty was 64 and had always been what she called 'a small sort', never quite reaching 5 ft. She had not had any trouble with her back before, but now she had a sudden, sharp pain in the thoracic region – that is, the part where the ribs come off. The pain extended right round to the front, on her left side, and prevented her bending or moving.

Her niece drove Kirsty home at snail's pace and called the doctor. Kirsty was in pain either standing up or sitting. The only relief she got was lying down. Even then she had an unpleasant colicky pain in her abdomen, which her doctor called *ileus*. Her stomach was bloated and she could not bear the thought of food. Her doctor said he thought she might have had a little bleeding from the back which had irritated her abdomen. X-rays showed several crushed vertebrae, and one in particular. The immediate treatment consisted of painkillers of the non-steroidal anti-inflammatory group (NSAIDs), commonly used in arthritis and bone pain.

Kirsty's pain gradually lessened over the next eight weeks, but meanwhile her back movements were restricted. She had difficulty getting her shoes on – they had to be slip-ons, and it was out of the question to cut her toenails. Long-handled scissors were too difficult to operate. Calcium and vitamin D supplements, together with a rejig of her diet and, as she improved, of her lifestyle, enabled Kirsty to recover almost completely. She can never neglect her bones in the future.

Acute effects of fractured vertebrae (only some may occur)

- Pain in the area of the affected bone: localized, radiating round to the front on one side, or a complete girdle of pain.
- Tenderness to pressure: this is not felt over the bone itself but in the muscle which goes into spasm to protect the injured part.
- Localized swelling.
- Severe limitation of movement, especially bending, stooping and lifting.
- Abdominal colic.
- Loss of appetite, vomiting, fever.

Long-term effects

- Further fractures – in more than 85 per cent of those who have had one vertebral fracture.
- Loss of height of more than 10 cm (4 ins) over the next decade.
- Nerve root pain from the nipping of a nerve from the bone changes. Fortunately this is seldom persistent.
- Numbness or paralysis from a nipped nerve. This is uncommon and also not likely to last.

- Kyphosis: this is the medical term for an increase in the forward concave curvature of the spine in the chest area, caused by anterior wedge fractures. In the upper part this is responsible for the 'dowager's hump', the sharp forward bend commonly seen in older ladies.

Kyphosis, plus a shortened backbone, can have several ill-effects:

- Your chin may nearly rest on your breast bone, because your muscles get tired with the effort of pulling your head up.
- The chest, including the lungs, is constricted, which means that you become short of breath more easily than before.
- Because of the loss of height in your backbone your whole rib cage moves downwards and may catch uncomfortably against the wings of the hip bones and the rim of the pelvis.
- A propensity to develop hiatus hernia, with burps and discomfort in the chest after meals and lying down.
- Inability to lie flat with a curved back – although fortunately most of us prefer to sleep on our sides in a curved, foetal attitude anyway.
- There is less room for your abdomen so it bulges out forwards – although you are no fatter or heavier than before.
- Constipation secondary to this altered abdominal situation.
- Standing and walking upright become difficult and tiring.
- A near-panicky fear of falling may develop from having a body of a different shape and balance.

Depression with anxiety is not uncommon, and very understandable if you have become an inelegant shape, your back aches, and you feel alarmingly insecure when you go out. A careful choice of clothes and a stick to give you confidence walking will help and so, even more, will treatment for the low mood. It is worth asking for this, since your doctor may be afraid of offending you by suggesting it. In the very short term it is reassuring to know that lying down usually provides quick, if temporary, relief when your back is hurting or your muscles weary.

At least none of these tribulations is dangerous.

Evelyn

Evelyn had the misfortune to be involved in a serious road traffic accident in her early forties. She was not the driver but on the vulnerable 'sui-side', in the front passenger seat. She had a major fracture of her femur, the big thigh bone, which took many months to heal after plating, and took a major chunk out of her bone mass. Although she was able to walk, Evelyn was unable to manage as much weight-bearing exercise as she had done previously with tennis, squash and golf. She took up swimming enthusiastically – fun in itself but it did her bones no favours.

She was well into the danger area for osteoporosis, especially as she was naturally a thin, willowy type with no spare flesh in her youth and somewhat gaunt in her fifties. Fortunately, the new GP who took her on at this stage was both knowledgeable and conscientious, and after hearing her medical history he set her off on a comprehensive, lifestyle anti-osteoporosis course. This was rather against Evelyn's inclinations but she went along with it. At 60 she has a respectable bone mineral density reading and she has no sign in her X-rays of fractures or crushed vertebrae.

Hip fractures

These are potentially the most disabling and dangerous fractures caused by osteoporosis, and are common. If you are a white woman aged 50 in the US or the UK you stand an 18 per cent chance of having a hip fracture during your remaining life span. This is only 6 per cent if you are a man. (The equivalent figures for fractures of the vertebrae are 16 per cent and 5 per cent.) Four out of five hip fractures affect women and falls are a major risk factor where women fare badly. They have an increasing number of falls from age 45. Sixty is a critical age, and between 60 and 64 the number having falls jumps from one in five to one in three.

Fortunately only 5 to 6 per cent result in broken hips. It very much depends on how you fall – if the impact is directly on your hip, and especially if you are slim, there is little to protect the bone.

While women are at increasing risk of fractures from age 45, plateauing at 60, in men the age-related increase is delayed until 65, but after that there is less difference between the sexes. Seventy-five is the average age for a hip fracture in either sex in England, but this varies from country to country. In order of vulnerability, white women come top, then Asian women, Asian men and finally, with the strongest skeletons of all – black men. Scandinavians have a high prevalence of hip fracture, probably due to their geography depriving them of enough strong sunshine. An odd anomaly – among the Bantu in South Africa and the Maoris in New Zealand, unlike other races, males and females are equally susceptible to osteoporosis and age makes little difference.

Although it can happen without any apparent trigger, a hip fracture usually results from a fall – not from a great height, but from a standing position on level ground. While most people are caught by surprise by the accident, in a few there has been some pain on putting weight on that side for days or even a few weeks before.

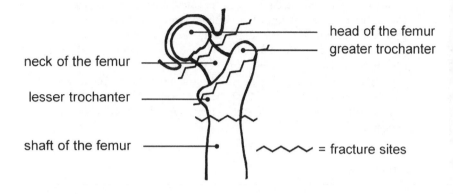

Immediate symptoms

- Pain in the hip: this can be severe or surprisingly mild, depending on the degree of trauma and blood loss.
- Inability to stand up: the problem is obvious from these two first symptoms.
- The leg is turned outwards.

An X-ray usually clinches the diagnosis, but sometimes, when the bones are not displaced, the break may not show up in a single film. Further X-rays may be needed.

Types of hip fracture

There are two main types of hip fracture: *trochanteric* and *cervical*, according to their position (see the diagram). Trochanteric fractures are also called *extracapsular* because they are right outside the actual joint and its covering. The cervical type are intracapsular, within the joint capsule. In either type the early symptoms are the same, but occasionally, with a cervical type, if the bones are impacted – a type of compression fracture – the victim can manage to hobble along and the diagnosis is not at first clear. The surgical part of the treatment depends on the site of the break and whether the bones are displaced (see p. 78).

Trochanteric breaks tend to occur in people about five years older than the cervical variety and the bone is more severely osteoporotic. Fragile trabecular bone which easily crumbles is mainly affected in these cases, while in the cervical type the hard outer bone is also involved.

14

Treatment

A hip fracture may turn out to be no more troublesome than a standard hip replacement for arthritis, and this operation is frequently carried out after a fracture. The treatment necessarily begins with a stay in hospital for surgery and pain relief, initially with powerful analgesics such as morphine (see p. 81 for details). Within 24 hours of the surgery a healthy-looking physiotherapist will be encouraging you to try standing up, and to your surprise you will find that you will be able to do it. From then on it is a matter of graded exercise, physiotherapy and medication, and if everything goes to plan you may be able to return home in four days.

Favourable circumstances

- Relative youth – that is, 75 or under.
- Trochanteric fracture – the lifetime chance of a second fracture is 8 per cent with this type, compared with 12 per cent after a cervical fracture.
- Sound mental and nervous health.
- Capable physically and psychologically of independent living before the fracture.

Longer-term results

Patience and persistence must be your watchwords. There is a 50/50 chance of getting back to all your accustomed activities within six months – but if not, persevere for another six months. It may easily take a year. Continuing pain is the commonest unwanted symptom, especially when standing or walking or with any of the activities below. Lack of energy – or rather, easy fatigue – is the second bugbear.

Tasks which may be difficult include:

- climbing stairs;
- getting on and off buses and trains and in and out of cars;
- housework, especially vacuuming;
- carrying, lifting, bending;
- shopping.

If you were not 100 per cent before the fracture, progress may be very slow.

There is also a 20 per cent risk of death in the first year, but not directly due to the fracture, and the danger falls off sharply from the second year onwards. Any other illnesses which are present are likely to get worse, not to recover, and in up to a third of cases there are complications from the surgery. They include delayed healing or failure of the bones to unite, degeneration of the head of the femur (see diagram), or pins and screws inserted may work loose. Keyhole surgery has improved the prognosis.

Oddly enough, complete hip replacement is less liable to problems than the partial operations often used in the very elderly. This is probably because patients are especially frail in the first place. It is tiresome to have to go through more treatment, but there is no situation which cannot be alleviated and none where you should stop trying. There is always a dividend.

Andrew

Andrew was 79. He had TB as a young man and after several stints in a sanatorium and the loss of part of his right lung, he was declared free from the tubercle bacillus. However, he was left without the physical resources to play sport, and his wife took over from his mother in cosseting more than was necessary. He was a 'net-head' at home and had done clerical work and later fixed computers for a living. All in all, the only outdoor exercise he took was the quick, guilty trip to the tobacconists. Of course he should never have smoked, but at the time he acquired the addiction people were not so clued up about the dangers.

Andrew had been retired for some years and felt as fit as ever he had – rather better, in fact – when he stumbled over his grandson's toy train on the bottom stair. He grabbed the banister but lost his balance and fell heavily on his right hip, his unlucky side. Not that he knew, but his bones were already brittle from osteoporosis, due to serious bone loss during his periods of illness and immobilization in early adulthood, the toxic effect of tobacco on bone formation, his relative lack of exercise and sunshine and his age – over 75.

It was a trochanteric fracture with severe disorganization of the crumbly bone, so the surgeon decided to go ahead with a hip replacement. It was a cold January, the peak period for fractured hips, and unfortunately Andrew developed a chest infection post-operatively. This meant that his rehabilitation programme was chequered and delayed. He was unable to walk without sticks for a full year, but his determination and courage, helped by his wife's support, finally paid off. He now walks for 20 minutes every day and takes calcium and one of the bisphosphonate medicines. He still enjoys surfing – the Net.

Colles' fracture

Abraham Colles was an eighteenth-century surgeon from Dublin. He was the first to describe a particular kind of fracture of the wrist caused by falling forwards on to the outstretched hand. It is especially common after the menopause and is one of the three fractures due to osteoporosis which affect 40 per cent of women at some time. The other two are hip and vertebral fractures. Fifteen per cent of women have a wrist fracture some time in their lives, with more than 20 per cent having had one or even two by age 70. One reason why women are affected so frequently is because of their greater propensity to falls compared with men.

The doctor's clinical examination of the injured wrist usually gives the diagnosis, and an X-ray will confirm it.

Symptoms

- Acute pain – the wrist can be more painful than a hip fracture.
- Tenderness.
- Swelling.
- Limitation of movement.
- The wrist is an odd shape.

The bones are displaced and require *reduction* under anaesthetic to correct their alignment. This tricky manoeuvre may have to be repeated more than once to get the position correct. The wrist and forearm are immobilized in plaster of Paris for four to six weeks and the bones usually unite well, but in a third of cases troublesome features, which may continue for months, are tenderness, swelling, stiffness and weakness – in the hand rather than the wrist. Occasionally a frozen shoulder develops.

Shoulder fracture

Fracture of the upper part of the humerus, the bone of the upper arm, is usually caused by the same type of fall as a Colles' fracture – forwards on to the outstretched hand. The victims are generally elderly – that is, over 75 – but they usually recover well with three or four weeks' simple immobilization, followed by physiotherapy for the muscles and the joint itself.

An alternative treatment is a *hemiarthroplasty* – replacing the round head of the bone, a little like a hip replacement. This provides a working joint almost at once, and is more satisfactory than trying to fix the joint with screws. As in all the cases of fracture due to osteoporosis, a medication, eating and exercise regimen must continue indefinitely afterwards.

Rita

Rita was 47. Both her mother and her grandmother had suffered from osteoporosis, but they had been old. Rita felt their problems were not relevant to her, so much younger. She still remembered her grandmother as a tiny, shrunken, little figure, bowed right over, walking very slowly with a stick. She died from pneumonia at 85, a good age for those days. Rita's mother had broken her wrist in a fall when she was

70, but Rita felt this was an accident which could happen to anyone. Her own main health problem, she believed, was her diabetes, the type requiring insulin injections.

Rita's fracture happened in the most unexpected circumstances – on a slippery dance floor. She and her partner somehow got their feet entangled and overbalanced, laughing. Rita found she could not get up and that she had an agonizing pain in her ankle. Six weeks in a walking plaster with calcium and a biphosphonate to slow down the rate of bone resorption (removal) allowed the bone to mend.

From the first X-ray it was clear that Rita had osteoporosis. It was in her genes and made worse by the diabetes. In her later forties, her oestrogen level was dipping sharply – a major factor in the development of brittle bones. Rita was consoled to read that she was in a similar situation to Prince Charles's wife, the Duchess of Cornwall – whose mother and grandmother had severe osteoporosis. If she – Rita – took the care her doctor advised, she could put this one fracture behind her and look forward to an active, healthy, interesting life.

3

Types of osteoporosis

The essence of osteoporosis comprises weak, brittle bones, liable to break at the slightest trauma. There are several routes to this end result, with two which are particularly important. One is directly related to the hormonal changes of the menopause and the other is driven by your age. It matters that you should know which type you have, since there are different methods for dealing with each.

Type 1: Menopausal osteoporosis

Characteristics

- Age range: 51–70.
- Sex ratio, female to male: 6:1 (hormonal changes affect men too, but to a lesser extent and later).
- Loss of bone: rapid and severe.
- Bone mineral density (BMD): sharply reduced.
- Type of bone affected: mainly trabecular.
- Commonest sites: vertebrae (backbone), wrist and to a lesser extent ankle.
- Type of vertebral fracture: crush and collapse, with a loss of more than 25 per cent in the height of each affected bone.
- Jaws affected: leading to loss of teeth.
- Parathyroid hormone (controls level of calcium): reduced, producing less stimulus to bone turnover.
- Cause of Type 1 osteoporosis: deficiency of sex hormones, especially oestrogen, triggered by the menopause.
- Likeliest first warning: acute pain in the back as vertebrae give way, taking as long as six months to subside.

The sequence of events

Bone mass

The amount of solid bone material in your body reaches its all-time high at around 30, and from 35 begins to decline. Resorption begins to outstrip new bone formation, and with the normal rate of bone renewal from 35 to around 45 there is an overall loss of 0.3 per cent each year.

19

The menopause

Between the ages of 45 and 55 in women the ovaries go into retirement and give up producing sex hormones (the adrenal glands take over at a reduced rate). These hormones include oestrone, androstenone, testosterone, progesterone – and oestrogen. The drop in oestrogen level stimulates bone turnover, and the deficit between loss and build-up of bone with each cycle leads to an annual shortfall of 2 to 3 per cent. This accelerated rate of bone loss continues for between four and eight years after your periods have stopped, then settles back into the earlier, gentle rate. There is, temporarily, a flood of calcium into the system from bone resorption, and this shows up in urine and blood tests.

All this is normal, since all women go through the change, but it does not amount to osteoporosis.

Genetic predisposition

This and probably other factors not yet identified lead to the development of Type 1 osteoporosis in 10 to 20 per cent of women in reaction to the menopause. The phase of rapid bone loss is likely to continue for 15 to 20 years in this group and is more severe. This is due to an extra large number of osteoclasts, the cells geared to disposing of old bone, while the osteoblasts, those in charge of bone-building, seem to function half-heartedly.

Vitamin D

The slight increase in parathyroid hormone inhibits the manufacture of this vitamin in your skin. If it is in short supply your intestine cannot properly absorb the calcium in your food. The end result is a low BMD and an enhanced risk of osteoporosis.

Angela

Angela was a healthy countrywoman, who included plenty of dairy products in her diet and whose work took her outdoors. She kept bees as a hobby and an extra source of income. Her periods petered out when she was 46, a little earlier than the average – and she was glad to be rid of the bother. Her forty-eighth birthday fell on a sunny day in August, when she planned to harvest some of the honey from her hive. She was using a smoker to make the bees drowsy, but one of them got inside her veil. In trying to cope with it she caught her foot on one of the legs of the hive. She put out her hand to save herself and fell on it quite heavily, jarring the bone on the thumb side of her forearm.

She knew she had done some damage because her wrist hurt so much – wrist fractures are particularly painful – and it quickly began to swell. An X-ray at the hospital showed a break in the radius, one of the forearm bones, with the upper end overriding the lower part: a typical Colles' fracture. The orthopaedic surgeon was unable to make the two parts stay together accurately by simple manipulation, so she had recourse to an external fixation device. This involved steel pins in the shaft of the radius and the metacarpals (hand bones) to keep the broken parts in position.

When the bone had mended, a few weeks later – checked by X-ray – the pins were removed. In most cases a little physiotherapy would have restored her wrist to normal, but Angela was one of the one-third of Colles' fracture sufferers who have ongoing problems. She continued to have mild twinges of pain, a stiff wrist and fingers and a poor grip. She also had *causalgia*, a curious tingling, burning sensation, usually due to irritation of a nerve.

Over the next nine months these symptoms gradually disappeared, but this wrist and hand have remained weaker than the other one. HRT was considered an essential part of Angela's treatment but not nowadays.

Natural history

Type 1 osteoporosis goes through a pattern of illness similar to that of asthma, rheumatoid arthritis and inflammatory bowel disease, among other conditions. These are long-term disorders that do not affect everyone, but in which the symptoms show up early on. Type 1 contrasts with Type 2, in this respect.

Type 2: Age-related osteoporosis

Characteristics

- Age range: 70 and over.
- Sex ratio, female to male: 2:1.
- Bone loss: less rapid and severe than in Type 1.
- BMD: only a little lower than the average for your age.
- Type of bone affected: cortical 50 to 70 per cent (not less than 50 per cent), trabecular 30 to 50 per cent.
- Sites of fracture: hip, vertebrae, also pelvis, shoulder, upper shin bone.
- Type of hip fracture: usually cervical – there is more cortical bone in the neck of the femur than between the trochanters (see diagram on p. 14).
- Type of vertebral fracture: group of wedge fractures of vertebrae at mid-chest level; loss of height of individual bones less than 25 per cent.
- Jaws and teeth not involved.

- The osteoblasts function poorly, worse than in Type 1, so bone formation is impaired greatly.
- Cause of Type 2 osteoporosis: a build-up of age-related changes leading to bone loss – basically a fall-off in bone formation compared with resorption. Age-related bone loss runs at an equal rate for both men and women from the age of 75 to 80, but women have a head start with the menopause.
- Characteristic signs and symptoms: insidious development of marked loss of height, and kyphosis with dowager's hump – back bent and head poked forward.

Natural history

Type 2 osteoporosis progresses according to the Gompertzian pattern (described by Ben Gompertz, a British actuary). The illness starts earlier than you realize, almost imperceptibly, and develops very gradually, producing symptoms late in life – it may never cause a clear-cut attack. It happens in a similar way to pouring water into a glass: nothing happens for a long time, but if the water reaches the brim it spills over. Most people develop some degree of Type 2 osteoporosis in their senior years, but there may be no definite warning incident.

Important effects of ageing

- Increased production of parathyroid hormone, stimulating bone turn-over, in turn leading to loss of bone substance.
- Impaired bone formation by the osteoblasts so that bone that is resorbed is not adequately replaced.
- Deficiency of vitamin D because of lack of exposure to sunlight for many old people, especially those who are housebound or live in homes for the elderly, and also because of impaired absorption in the intestine of vitamin D in the diet.
- Inadequate absorption of calcium because of the shortage of vitamin D.
- Postmenopausal oestrogen deficiency adds to the bone loss.

There is a good deal of overlap between Type 1 and Type 2 osteoporosis, and some people have a mixture of both sets of symptoms.

Geoffrey

Geoffrey was 84 when he broke his hip. He had been an active man in his youth and had broken his collarbone at rugby and his shin bone in a motorbike accident. Now he lived in a flat near the city centre and could not raise any enthusiasm for taking a walk. His greatest pleasure was in smoking his pipe and having a whisky – or two – in the evenings. He sometimes went to his club for same plus a chinwag with his old pals.

Geoffrey's break was in the neck of the thigh bone, but the bone was so fragile that there was no possibility of pinning it. The hip replacement was a success, although he had to remain in hospital for three weeks while it healed. Geoffrey did not mind taking regular calcium and vitamin D, and the calcitonin which should theoretically be helpful for men with osteoporosis. He did not really object to being chivvied by the physiotherapist into doing a boring set of exercises most days and struggling to walk increasing distances with two sticks and then only one.

What did get to him was the orthopaedic surgeon's veto on alcohol and tobacco – which he said had contributed to Geoffrey's fracture, and would continue to damage his bone structure if he continued. His GP and his wife support the surgeon, so Geoffrey is outnumbered and – as they keep telling him – at least he has had no further disasters in the last ten months.

Juvenile osteoporosis

Bone development is at its most rapid in infancy and adolescence; at least half the peak bone mass is acquired in the second decade. This is money in the bone bank, a nest-egg for contingencies. Its size is largely – 60 to 80 per cent – decided by your genes, but it can only reach its full potential if, especially during your adolescent growth spurt, you have liberal, properly balanced nourishment, a well-developed body, including the appropriate production of sex hormones, and a healthy lifestyle with plenty of exercise and open air.

Children and adolescents need much more calcium than is generally available in the diet of most of the world's population, and more than the level still considered adequate in some 'first world' countries.

- Children require 1200 mg daily.
- 11–24 year olds need 1500 mg daily.

These are the amounts recommended by the National Osteoporosis Society of the UK, and they are more than double what the Department of Health suggests. Experts in the USA agree with the NOS.

Osteoporosis in childhood can develop before birth. Premature babies lose out on the bone mass they would have acquired in their last three months in the womb. Fortunately, if all goes well, they achieve a normal bone mineral density (BMD) by the age of one or two years, and are at no special risk of brittle bones later. Turner's syndrome (a chromosomal disorder that affects the whole body), cystic fibrosis, and any illness treated with big doses of steroids, or, more simply, a lack of calcium and vitamin D in the diet – all correlate with a low bone mass in a youngster, and the risk of osteoporosis.

Since childhood and adolescence are dynamic periods for growth there can be 'catch-up' periods in the amount of bone (bone mass) and its strength – with adequate supplies of the raw materials. The long-term results need be nothing to fear, even after a fracture from osteoporosis.

Anorexia nervosa, slimming and excessive exercise

Anorexia nervosa is a psychosomatic plague affecting adolescent girls. The starvation diet they go in for leads to a lack of female hormones and, inevitably, no periods. If the condition lasts for many months, even years, the situation is like the menopause. A shortage of oestrogen, plus very poor nutrition, can lead to osteoporosis with fractures – before the age of 20!

Recovery from the abnormal eating pattern can still leave the bones depleted of minerals and brittle, and the bone mass reduced – long term. Energetic treatment is essential: a super-nourishing diet with calcium and vitamin D, psychological treatment to get the girl to eat it, and in some cases oestrogen therapy.

Slimming bouts which stop short of the persistence of anorexia can also have deleterious effects on the bones, in adult women as well as adolescents. Osteoporosis can cause bones to break without adequate cause in these cases, too.

Serious training for ballet or athletics can involve excessive amounts of physical exercise. In females this can switch off the sex hormones and bring the periods to a halt – with a devastating effect on the BMD and the reserves in the bone bank. Less exercise and more food are needed to reduce the risk of broken bones, but, as with anorexia nervosa, an ambitious youngster may be uncooperative. It is a matter of endless patience by the parents and therapist, and for them to weigh up the value of athletic success compared with risks to health.

Svetlana

Svetlana's mother had been a prima ballerina and at 16 she was at ballet school herself, burning with determination to do equally well. The training was hard and she put everything into it, and she was also anxious to keep her weight low enough for the male dancers to lift her easily. Without realizing, she slipped into an anorexic regime, allowing herself a maximum of 600 calories daily. Her periods consisted of two or three token bleeds spaced out during her fifteenth year, after which they stopped altogether.

It certainly was not her fault that the male student dropped her, but her brittle arm bones were a direct result of her lifestyle. Her shoulder was slow to mend because of the fragility of the bone and her low calcium intake. She avoided dairy foods as fattening, almost panicking at the sight of a glass of milk. The principal of the ballet school, to whom this was an all too familiar picture, suspended Svetlana from her studies until she should have reached an agreed target weight and her BMD showed signs of improvement.

Svetlana is still struggling, but she now clocks eight stone and has had one light period. She has not taken any extra oestrogen, but eats a generous allowance of nutritious foods, including all the natural sources of calcium.

Pregnancy, breastfeeding and osteoporosis

Your body is so adaptable that normally it can take in its stride the provision of minerals to a foetus while at the same time protecting your own bones from being depleted. Pregnancy produces a huge flow of oestrogen which in turn leads to these bodily adjustments. Your gut plays its part by absorbing twice as much calcium as usual, so long as your diet provides it; and the concentration of vitamin D increases from 15–60 pg to 80–100 pg/ml. The result is that, in a normal pregnancy, you lose no bone minerals, and some women actually increase their bone reserve.

This is just as well, if you mean to feed your baby yourself.

Twins are a special case: a double drain on their mother's bones, more liable to prematurity than singletons, and more at risk of osteoporosis at some stage in their lives.

Breastfeeding

This is a drain on the mother's bone bank. Breastfeeding for six months means a 7 per cent loss of bone mass, but this can recover fully by the time the baby is 18 months old, so long as the feeding does not go on much past the sixth month.

Throughout pregnancy and breastfeeding, 1500 mg of calcium daily is needed. If this falls short osteoporosis may develop. You might think that women who have never had children would be less likely to have osteoporosis in later life – not so! Elderly women (65-plus) who produced several children earlier in their lives tend to have a higher BMD than those with none. The exception is teenage pregnancy. It puts too great a strain on the mother's body, still growing, and this is reflected in weaker bones – still – at 65.

Osteoporosis associated with pregnancy

This comes in two types, both of which are rare.

- *Transient osteoporosis of the hip.* This crops up in the last three months of the pregnancy, causing pain in the hip and groin, but no frank break. The bone recovers its strength with adequate treatment, but the pain may linger on.

- *Spinal osteoporosis*. This only occurs after a first baby, within three months of the birth. The effect is vertebral compression, causing a loss of height and pain in the back. The bone mass recovers, and there is no risk of a recurrence with another pregnancy.

Osteoporosis in men

Men are the lucky ones – they have a very much lower risk of osteoporosis than women. But they are not immune, and when they do develop the disease it is six times as likely to be the age-related Type 2 as the hormonal variety. Bone loss due to ageing alone takes a long time to lead to a fracture. Since men have a shorter life span, some of them never reach the critical level of loss where a bone break is on the cards.

Up to age 44, men suffer many more broken bones than women because of their lifestyle, but somewhere between 40 and 50 the ratio switches and from then on women greatly outnumber men in the fracture stakes. Nevertheless, men's bones, like women's, become more fragile from mid-life onwards. Hip and spine fractures are the commonest. The broken bones of earlier life – from sport and accident – do leave a legacy of reduced bone mass, making fractures from minimal-to-moderate injury more likely. This applies especially to the hip. No one knows why, but these fractures are escalating more steeply in men than women, and carry a greater risk of death (still a minority).

Vertebral fractures in men cause loss of height and kyphosis, as in women, with an increased risk of further breaks. As for hip fractures in the over-75s, only half as many men as women suffer from this type.

Men have built-in advantages – larger, stronger skeletons, providing a more substantial bone mass from the outset; and no dramatic fall-off in sex hormones equivalent to the menopause. This means that a man who develops osteoporosis is more likely to have a secondary cause for it, for instance a chronic illness, diabetes, alcoholism, tobacco addiction, liver disease, operations on the stomach and the use of various drugs and medicines.

Low levels of male sex hormone tend towards osteoporosis by similar mechanisms to oestrogen deficiency. The causes of *hypogonadism* (underactive sexual organs) are developmental, associated with the genetic disorders Klinefelter's and Kallmann's diseases, operations on the testicles for cancer, and accidental injuries. A late puberty can have a knock-on effect, leading to a lower than normal level of sex hormone indefinitely. In these cases treatment includes androgens (male sex hormones, such as testosterone), a parallel to HRT (oestrogen and progesterone in women).

George

George was 62 and saw himself as fit and strong. It was on a Sunday afternoon in October when he was digging in the garden that a sharp pain in his back took his breath away. His wife drove him to the local Accident and Emergency Department, where an X-ray showed that he had a wedge fracture in the vertebra on a level with his tenth rib. The doctor gave him some painkillers at the hospital and his GP continued them, and also suggested either ice-packs or hot packs, whichever suited him best. These ploys helped him moderately well, but three weeks later his back still hurt him when he was walking or standing. He could not get on with his ordinary life.

Some two or three years before, he had slipped on the edge of an icy kerb and broken his wrist, and to all intents and purposes this had healed satisfactorily – but inevitably leaving a bone deficit. He was a moderate smoker and drinker – two packs a day and two drinks – and his work was sedentary. A thorough physical examination showed no other disease and, specifically, no particular reason for him to suffer from falls, the common cause of fractures. George's treatment involved an overhaul of his lifestyle, with extra calcium and vitamin D; regular, vigorous, weight-bearing exercise (but avoiding bending forwards); a course of physiotherapy – and dumping the cigarettes.

4

Secondary osteoporosis

1 Due to medication or other drugs

Osteoporosis may arise secondarily to the effects of a drug, usually given as medication. The most important of these conditions is the result of the ubiquitous, effective steroid medicines.

Steroid-induced osteoporosis

In 1932 the American neurologist Harvey Cushing was studying the adrenal gland, and discovered that a class of steroid compounds called *glucocorticoids* could cause osteoporosis. He was working with nature's own steroid, cortisol, which is produced in excess in Cushing's disease. By the 1940s it was realized that steroids given as medicines had the same devastating effect. This was noticed first with sufferers from rheumatoid arthritis. This was understandable since the illness itself induces some thinning of the bones, making them particularly susceptible to full-blown osteoporosis from other causes. A number of patients given the new, almost magical steroid medication developed compression fractures of their vertebrae.

Vertebral fractures are usually the first manifestation of steroid osteoporosis, although the hip and the long bones in the limbs may also be affected.

Who gets steroid-induced osteoporosis?

Almost anyone! The term osteoporosis automatically conjures up the stereotype of a little, bent old lady with a dowager's hump, hobbling along with a stick because of a hip fracture. In the case of steroid osteoporosis this is way off beam. Everyone who takes glucocorticoid steroids for six months develops some degree of osteoporosis, and it can crop up much sooner. Since these medicines are used in a wide range of illnesses, from chronic airways disease to sarcoidosis to Crohn's disease, it stands to reason that an equally wide range of people are subject to this type of osteoporosis.

They include men as well as women, children as well as young adults and seniors, black people as well as whites and Asians, and – for women – those who have had children and those who have had none. It makes no odds which illness it is – the effect of the medication on the bones is the same. Although high doses increase the risk, some people, especially men, are affected by quite low doses. In fact, within a few hours of a single dose of prednisolone, a frequently used steroid medicine, routine replacement of old, worn-out bone comes to a halt.

How steroids undermine your bones

- Severe, direct inhibitory effect on the osteoblasts, the cells responsible for bone-building.
- The activity of the bone-destroying osteoclasts is stimulated.
- The absorption of calcium from the gut is reduced, regardless of the availability of vitamin D.
- Parathyroid hormone levels are increased, leading to more rapid bone turnover with a further loss of minerals.
- Sex hormone production – in either sex – is suppressed, contributing to the loss of bone, as with the menopause.
- The kidneys let more calcium escape in the urine, leaving less for the bones.

Ploys to reduce the risk of osteoporosis with steroids

Begin these measures as soon as you start on the medication, with your doctor's help and say-so, and within the limits of what you can do.

- Whenever possible, use steroids you can inhale, as in asthma, or apply to your skin, as in dermatitis – instead of swallowing tablets or having injections.
- Keep to the lowest dose that is effective.
- Take the medication on alternate days, to give your bones a rest from the drug – the dose will be larger.
- Use short-acting rather than long-acting preparations for the same reason – to give your bones brief respite between doses.
- Keep your muscles both strong and big by whatever exercise your illness allows you to do. Get your physiotherapist's advice about specific exercises for the thigh, shoulder and trunk muscles in particular.
- Take 1500 mg of calcium daily.
- Cut down on salt.
- Take male hormone if you are a man with a low testosterone level.
- Have bone mass or BMD assessments every six months for the first two years after starting steroids, then review.
- Take calcitonin or another anti-osteoporosis medicine if rapid bone loss continues for several weeks.

Bryony

Bryony was 60. She had suffered from polymyalgia rheumatica for ten years and the only treatment that had helped her was prednisolone. She had now been taking it for eight years and had developed the 'moon face' that is typical of long-term steroids. Her doctor was concerned and arranged for BMD estimations. These were very low, showing Bryony to be in imminent danger of a fracture in her back or hip. The doctor was adamant that she must reduce her dose of prednisolone, currently running at 10 mg daily, but each time she tried her limbs became too stiff and painful for her to walk properly.

The next ploy was to try a snail's-pace reduction of 1 mg per month, backed up by calcium and multivitamins, including vitamin D. Bryony had more pain and no energy and fell into low spirits. It was at this point that the GP prescribed a two-week course of etidronate, to be repeated every three months. It has a particularly good reputation for bone pain and it helped Bryony. It is too early to judge, because this is a slow-acting treatment, but she does feel a little better in herself.

Alcohol

There is a general consensus among the experts that two drinks a day does no harm to the bones, a moderate intake is equivocal, while heavy drinking is extremely damaging. Ten per cent of men who suffer back fractures are found to abuse alcohol.

Ill-effects of alcohol on the bones

- Directly toxic to the osteoblasts, making for less bone renewal.
- Liver disease, causing increased bone turnover.
- Reduced levels of testosterone.
- Disturbed nutrition, with protein lack and sometimes general malnourishment.
- Poor absorption of vitamin D and calcium.
- Often weight loss and becoming unduly thin.
- Risk of falls increased.

Men are more liable to drink too much but this does not usually cause osteoporosis before the age of 60. From 60 to 69 the numbers escalate dramatically. Middle-aged women quite often emerge as secret – or discreet – heavy drinkers, and as they are already more susceptible to osteoporosis due to their sex, they may develop the disorder from their forties onwards. In addition, people who use alcohol too generously are likely to have a lifestyle involving smoking, coffee-drinking and too little exercise.

Tobacco

The adverse effects of smoking develop slowly but inexorably, with as few as ten cigarettes a day, and ultimately cause symptoms of osteoporosis. This is usually a fracture of the spine, hip or forearm, in the over-75 age group, when the protective function for the bones of body fat and oestrogen has greatly declined.

How tobacco can harm your bones

- Brings the start date of the menopause forward.
- Increases the likelihood of being thin.
- Less body weight, meaning less stimulus to bone-building.
- Increased bone resorption.
- Decreased bone formation – adding up to bone loss.
- Breaking down of natural oestrogen and also when it is given as HRT.
- Lifestyle likely to be as for alcohol.

Bone mass in smokers of either sex drops to the level of a person 40 years older.

Thyroxine

An excess of this hormone can come about through the disease of thyrotoxicosis, but is more likely to arise from over-enthusiastic treatment of an underactive thyroid, a common condition in middle-aged women. Recent research in the USA showed that 80 per cent of those treated for hypothyroidism were receiving excessive doses.

Thyroxine causes increased frequency of the activation of the bone turnover cycle, with reduced bone mineral density and the risk of osteoporosis.

Anticonvulsants

Osteomalacia, the adult form of rickets, due to a shortage of vitamin D, has long been associated with the drugs given for epilepsy, dating from the days when sufferers often lived in institutions and had very little opportunity of going outside. Nowadays they are more likely to develop osteoporosis.

High doses and a mixture of several anti-epileptic medicines in an elderly person who sees too little sunlight is the worst case scenario. These drugs break down vitamin D, leading to a harmful shortage in older people.

Anti-sex hormone drugs

These hormone medicines are used in premenstrual tension (PMT), endometriosis, polycystic ovaries and prostate cancer. They cause bone loss by speeding up the turnover. The anti-oestrogen drug, tamoxifen, used to prevent or control breast cancer has a mixed role, part harmful, part helpful to the bones.

People taking mood stabilizers or major tranquillizers long term are at increased risk of developing osteoporosis. The mechanism is hormonal. These drugs, of which the longest established are chlorpromazine and haloperidol, increase the production of prolactin, causing hyperprolactinaemia. This causes a reduction in the level of the sex hormones, testosterone in men and oestrogen in women, leading in turn to a loss of bone strength and osteoporosis. Men are affected more than postmenopausal women.

Because patients with schizophrenia frequently require continuous use of the tranquillizing medication, osteoporosis is linked with the illness, and also with other disorders for which this medication is used. The manic phase of bipolar affective illness is one such.

Heparin

This is an anti-clotting agent used in heart and artery disease and thrombophlebitis – clotting in a vein. It is often used in pregnancy for recurrent thrombophlebitis, since the other common anticoagulant, warfarin, can cause abnormalities in the unborn baby. Heparin stimulates the osteoclasts to break down more bone, and if used for six months or more will cause osteoporosis.

Lithium

This medicine, used long term in some psychiatric disorders, stimulates the production of parathyroid hormone which in turn accelerates the rate of bone loss from the normal cycle. BMD is reduced and the danger of osteoporosis goes up.

Methotrexate and other cytotoxic medicines

These drugs are used in leukaemia, lymphoma and several cancers. They inhibit new growth – including the formation of new bone.

Vitamin D

Excess of this vitamin has the reverse effect to that intended. It causes toxicity and if the excess is prolonged it leads to osteoporosis.

Medication likely to increase the risk of falls

- Sleeping tablets.
- Tablets for anxiety.
- Tranquillizers for more serious conditions.
- Diabetic medicines to reduce the blood sugar.
- Drugs to lower the blood pressure.
- Digoxin and some other heart medicines.
- Some powerful water tablets of the 'loop' type.

And alcohol.

2 Associated with some other chronic disease

Fifty per cent of those sustaining a hip fracture have some other chronic condition apart from osteoporosis, but since most of these people are over 70, this is not very surprising. Any restriction on exercise – due to illness – increases the likelihood of osteoporosis.

Disorders causing increased breakdown (resorption) and build-up (formation) of bone – with a net loss:

- thyrotoxicosis – overactive thyroid;
- Paget's disease of the bones.

Those causing increased resorption and decreased bone formation:

- rheumatoid arthritis, including the juvenile form;
- multiple sclerosis.

Those causing lack of calcium:

- kidney disease;
- intolerance to milk products (lactase deficiency).

Illnesses that can be beneficial:

- severe osteoarthritis of the hip – making fracture of the neck of the femur less likely;
- non-insulin dependent diabetes in women: the tendency to fat means more oestrogen, fewer falls and less damage if you do fall.

Rheumatoid arthritis

The danger of a hip fracture is doubled, and that for a crushed vertebra also increased. You are likely to take steroids with this disease, which increases the risk. Generalized bone thinning may also occur if you use non-steroidal anti-inflammatory drugs – NSAIDs – only.

Digestive system diseases

Coeliac disease, ulcerative colitis, Crohn's disease, and stomach operations for ulcers all lead to an inability to absorb properly essential nourishment, minerals and vitamins. Osteoporosis can result.

Luke

Luke was 17 when he developed Crohn's disease, the most serious of the inflammatory bowel diseases and the one most likely to be associated with osteoporosis. A few years after the initial diagnosis he ran into a bad patch and the upshot was an operation to remove an affected part of his intestine – *ileal resection*. He was also given steroids.

The disease and the loss of part of his gut meant that his absorption was impaired even for the normal nutrients – proteins, fats and carbohydrates, and also the calcium, vitamin D and magnesium he needed. He became very thin, which increased the risk of osteoporosis into the bargain. Blood tests revealed abnormally low levels of vitamin D, and BMD estimation showed his bones to be depleted and osteoporotic.

Luke did not have a fracture but his bones ached deeply and he was generally weak at an age when he should have been strong. The symptoms subsided with large doses of vitamin D, plenty of dairy products plus a calcium supplement, and winding down the steroid.

Some other diseases which may be associated with osteoporosis

- Haemophilia.
- Severe liver disease.
- Insulin-dependent diabetes.
- Sarcoidosis.
- Thalassaemia.
- Pernicious anaemia.
- Idiopathic scoliosis.
- Overactive thyroid.
- Cystic fibrosis.
- Acromegaly.
- Obstructive airways disease.
- Ankylosing spondylitis.
- Leukaemia, lymphoma, myeloma, breast and some other cancers.
- Lung cancer, which has a particular reputation for being associated with osteoporosis in men.
- Parkinson's disease.
- Various genetic disorders, mostly rare, such as osteogenesis imperfecta.

5

The risks

Are you living dangerously? It may be exhilarating to risk life and limb on a ski slope or racing at Brands Hatch, but there is no fun in putting your body at risk from osteoporosis.

The risk factors from this potentially crippling disease come in two packs: those you can do nothing about and the ones you can avoid or modify. You need to know about the first type, those which are out of your control, just as much as the second lot. If you were setting off on a long trip into the unknown, you would want to know of any faults or weaknesses in your equipment. On your life journey, similarly, it is important to know the weak spots for you.

Risk factors 1: Unavoidable

Sex

All along the line, women lose out in the osteoporosis stakes. Even before the menopause, their bones are lighter and less strong, and from 45 or so, when the female hormones go into reduced production, there is a dramatic – six-fold – difference between men and women in the prevalence of osteoporosis and its major symptom – easily broken bones. Even in grand old age, twice as many women as men have hip fractures.

Age

There is no fooling yourself that age does not signify. Your mind may be Mensa-sharp, your contours sylph-like and even your face lifted to a facsimile of youth, but your bones know precisely how old they are and they function accordingly – slowly shedding mineral strength from age 30 onwards. By the age of 80, 70 per cent of white women in the US and UK have osteoporosis and all but 3 per cent of the rest have osteopenia – lightweight bones. People used to think that from about 85 the rhythm of resorption and formation was ticking over so slowly that there was no further bone loss. In fact you go on losing bone density right into your nineties and onwards. There is never a time when you can take your bones for granted.

Your bones are under extra strain in early childhood and adolescence, when they are growing fast, and for women during the hormonal revolution of the menopause – and in the senior years, for everyone.

Late puberty in either sex, and an early menopause in women, lead to reduced bone mass – a major risk factor. Men do not have such a sharp shut-down of sex hormone production, but by 60 to 65 their bones, too, become more vulnerable. Every year from this age on, whichever your sex, you have to be more on your guard against the danger of a fracture.

Race

Wherever you now live, your bones will remember their ancestry. People of black African descent, especially men, are the most resistant to osteoporosis, and Asian men are the next luckiest. Women of almost all races are more susceptible than the men of the same race. White Caucasian women – the majority in North America and Northern Europe – stand the least chance of getting through life without osteoporosis, unless they take bone-care seriously. White people, across the board, have twice as many fractures from osteoporosis as those from African and Asian backgrounds. Hispanic Americans score midway between whites and blacks for susceptibility.

A few races buck the trend. Among the Malays and Chinese, men are more liable to osteoporosis than women, and it is more or less evens for the Bantu and the Maoris. These last two have very much less trouble with their bones than people of European descent living in the same region.

Where you live

Although race has a major influence, the country you live in is also important. Black men and women who have lived for several generations in the States and have absorbed the Western lifestyle have more osteoporosis than their cousins in Africa – although still much less than the whites.

The league table – from places with the largest proportion with osteoporosis down to the least – is as follows:

- Northern Europe/Scandinavia
- North America
- Asia
- South Pacific
- Southern Europe
- Africa

In Sweden and other countries in northern latitudes, the sun in winter is so low in the sky that there is a lot of the atmosphere for its rays to penetrate, and much of the ultraviolet does not get through. This interferes with the beneficial effect of sunlight on the manufacture of vitamin D. Vitamin D deficiency is common in these countries, all the more since so few foods provide it (basically only fish liver oil and egg yolk). There is much more osteoporosis in northern Europe than on the sunny Mediterranean coast. Similarly, in Britain there are more cases in Aberdeen than in Bournemouth – but perhaps this is partly due to more oatmeal in the Scottish diet – porridge and oatcakes – inhibiting the absorption of calcium, and whisky impeding new bone formation.

When there is less UV light, black and brown people are the likeliest to suffer from vitamin D deficiency. It is not by chance that Scandinavians are pale-skinned and blond, while those from sunny Spain and Italy have olive complexions.

One geographical quirk – the number of new cases of osteoporosis per year has levelled out in the US, but is still escalating in the UK, Sweden, Hong Kong and Australia.

Personal

Your family

Apart from the broad brush strokes of race, your personal heredity from the family makes a big difference. If one of your parents or another first-degree relative has osteoporosis you could be in line for it – a mother–daughter hand-on is the commonest. Identical twins start with a similar peak bone mass, but this can be blurred later by the effects of smoking, alcohol or other differences in lifestyle.

Your physique

This may be a racial or family trait, or due to early nutrition, but if you are smaller than average and lightly built you may be at greater risk. A hunky black man will have a substantial bone mass to fall back on – you will have less insurance. However, some small, slight Chinese and Japanese people have bones which are just as dense and strong as those of the big guys.

Other factors

- *Being a twin* leads to a lower bone mass.
- *No kids* by the time you have hit the menopause leaves you with a slightly lower bone mass and a slightly increased chance of osteoporosis.
- *Lactase deficiency* (in your genes) or some other cause for an inability to tolerate dairy foods, rich in calcium, is a big disadvantage.

Medical history – negative factors

- Periods irregular or missing, showing a shortage of oestrogen.
- Accidents involving broken bones, causing a reduction of bone mass.
- Operations on your stomach or intestines leading to poor absorption of calcium and vitamin D from food.

- Hysterectomy with removal of the ovaries, with a dramatic fall in oestrogen production.
- Hysterectomy without removal of the ovaries, leading to a temporary reduction in oestrogen (sometimes permanent) and bringing forward the start of the menopause.
- Sterilization by tying the tubes, which also reduces oestrogen level.
- Prostate or testicle surgery, leading to loss of male hormone.
- Chronic illnesses, particularly those involving immobilization or inhibition of new bone formation, for instance cancers.

Risk factors 2: Those you may be able to influence

- Caffeine – in excess.
- Tobacco – at all.
- Alcohol – more than one drink a day. Coffee, ciggies and booze are enemies which can feel like friends – a pleasure, a comfort, but more especially a habit.
- Sedentary lifestyle or enforced inactivity because of illness or handicap.
- Diet which impairs the absorption of calcium, for example
  – wheat bran, beans and wholemeal, containing phytates;
  – spinach and rhubarb, because of oxalates (see p. 108);
  – too much protein and sodium, causing loss of calcium in the urine;
  – fast foods and other processed foods low in calcium and high in phosphate and sodium content.
- Shortage of vitamins K, C and D.
- Lack of trace elements – zinc, manganese, magnesium, copper (see also Chapter 14 on diet).
- Contraceptive pill – maybe: it seems to have an effect either way, reducing or increasing the BMD.
- Not taking hormone replacement therapy after the menopause, although HRT also has dangers.
- Poorly developed muscles.
- Radiotherapy and chemotherapy.
- Medicines interfering with the absorption of calcium:
  – 'loop' water pills such as frusemide or triamterene;
  – tetracycline, an antibiotic;
  – anticonvulsants;
  – steroids;
  – antacids containing aluminium salts;
  – thyroxine;
  – isoniazid, used in TB.

Naomi

Emika and Naomi were friends, both working in London for a Japanese firm. Emika came from Tokyo, Naomi from Manchester. Both were 29, small and neat and weighing in at around 50 kg. Each thought the other was slightly slimmer and decided to reverse the situation. The result was a competition to see who could eat the least and lose the most. Both were determined characters and neither would give up. It went on for months, with Naomi dipping into anorexia – until the accident.

Naomi was keen on football, she thought it cool. When she fell on the ball and then the ground, her wrist broke. The X-ray in casualty revealed her thinned-out bones – she had osteoporosis. She was shocked to find she had an old ladies' disease, severe enough to show up on the film. She wondered why Emika, who had done exactly the same slimming, had no problem and a DEXA test (see p. 46) showed that her BMD was normal. The difference was that while Naomi's weight was low for an English girl, it was around average for a Japanese; and while Emika's periods continued as usual, Naomi's were on the blink, making her bones all the more vulnerable.

Naomi is now trying to rebuild her bones with extra calcium and vitamin D – and a good mixed diet.

Special risks for seniors

It behoves those of retirement age to be considerate of their bones, particularly with regard to falls. A third of their age group have at least one fall a year, of which 6 per cent result in a fracture. Three-quarters of falls which end fatally occur in those over 65 – and they are 99 per cent due to osteoporosis.

The propensity for falls

Causes include:

- Impaired sense of balance.
- Poor muscle control.
- Slow reaction time and weak muscles, so that you cannot save yourself.
- Drugs causing confusion and dizziness, especially sleeping tablets, tranquillizers, sedatives, and antidepressants (see also chapter 4).
- Alcohol.
- Low blood pressure, sometimes due to medicines given to reduce a high pressure.
- Unstable joints, especially the knees.

- Arthritis, either rheumatoid or osteoarthritis, affecting how you walk.
- Parkinson's disease.
- Impaired vision, hearing and balance organ in the ear (you may not hear traffic until it is very close).
- Foot problems – for instance, bunions, corns, callosities or overgrown toenails – affecting walking.

Low calcium level

- Calcium is less well absorbed by older people.
- Less use of dairy products in this group.
- Generally inadequate diet, especially among those living in homes for the elderly.

Other considerations

- Older people take less exercise.
- Fewer outdoor activities – and less ultraviolet light.
- Less response by the skin to sunlight – less vitamin D made.
- Depression of mood, poor memory – may forget to take supplements to diet.

Jessie

Jessie was 72. She had always been very concerned about her appearance, fretting miserably if she put on an extra pound on holiday. She kept her figure trim with diet, but not exercise: this was her first mistake. Walking exercise would have been difficult with the high heels she invariably wore – not quite stilettos, but near. She could not bear the thought of 'flat barges, like a yokel'. It was a nuisance to find her sight was not as good as it had been, but she did not want to wear glasses in public.

The final straw – not Jessie's fault – was the freezing. The pavement was like glass but she did not see it clearly when she slipped and fell crack on her hip. She did quite well with her hip replacement, but would have been walking better if her bones had been stronger. She is now doing daily exercises recommended by the physiotherapist, and is improving.

Safety net for seniors

- Precautions against falls: shock-absorbent flooring, no loose rugs, hand-grips for bath and stairs, good lighting, well-fitting shoes, hip protectors. Hip protectors, oddly, are most beneficial in institutions.
- Diet designed to include all necessary nutrients, vitamins and minerals.
- Supplements of calcium and vitamin D.

- Daily exercise schedule, preferably walking, but whatever you can manage: extra calcium does not make up for lack of weight-bearing muscular activity.
- Treatment for depression, if you are feeling low and without energy or interest.
- Review of medicines, with a view to cutting down or out any that are not now necessary.

6

Finding out: Diagnostic tests

Screening

Although thousands more women in the UK get osteoporosis than cancer of the cervix, regular smear tests are laid on for the latter, but there is nothing to check for osteoporosis. The object of screening is to find out if trouble is brewing, before there are any symptoms to alert you. Treatment at this stage can prevent serious problems later, but the essential first step is to find out how healthy your bones are now, and whether osteoporosis has already begun to set in.

Ideally every woman should be screened for osteoporosis when she has her menopause, usually at around 50, when the female sex hormones take a nosedive. Men who are fit and symptom-free can afford to delay another ten years before they enter the danger period, when they, too, are definitely at risk of osteoporosis. Do not wait for a bone to break, or to find that you are not as tall as you were because your vertebrae are slowly collapsing. Take action now to sidestep such nasties by anti-osteoporosis manoeuvres, before any serious damage has been done.

Unfortunately the NHS does not provide screening for osteoporosis for normal men and women in the risk areas of 60 and 45 respectively.

Is there a local scheme in your neighbourhood?

In my area the municipal swimming pool and health facility has taken the initiative by offering half-hour check-out sessions for osteoporosis, including an ultrasound examination for anyone who wants one. The snag is that you have to pay – and you do not even know whether you need a test. If you are already of retirement age it may be worth asking your GP to refer you via the NHS for ultrasound or one of the other new, sophisticated technological methods of examining the living bone.

If you come in for more than one or two of the risk factors reviewed in Chapter 5, tell your doctor. Of course, if you have had a wrist or hip fracture, have lost height or suffer from persistent backache, you definitely and urgently need to have an assessment of your bone mass or bone mineral density. To recap from Chapter 1, these two measures go hand in hand and are the best indicators we have of bone strength and the identification of osteoporosis. The lower the bone mass and BMD, the greater the risk of a fracture. Healthy bones do not break without being subjected to considerable force. Falling to the ground from a standing – or even sitting – position does not qualify, nor, of course, the long-term pressure on your spine of the weight of your body.

It struck me, as I wrote this, that I, personally, did not want to run any unnecessary risks. I decided to take up for myself the swimming pool offer.

My test

Eight years ago, I had to pay £39 up-front when I booked in. I wondered if I would have to undress, and made sure my undies were pristine. I need not have bothered. To start with, the two girls running the show, both under 25 and looking very fit, asked me my age, all about my periods from start to finish, my children and if I had breastfed them, whether anyone in the family had osteoporosis, my lifestyle including diet, exercise, cigarettes and alcohol, what medicines, if any, I was taking, any operations, especially gynaecological ones, and finally, any fractures. They noted that my periods had been irregular, and that five years ago I had broken my ankle, merely by turning round sharply in the street – an early warning if I had been more with it.

Then came the high spot – the ultrasound. I had to take off my shoes and socks and my heels were anointed with oil. I put each of them in turn in a kind of heel rest – briefly – and felt nothing. They gave me the answer immediately, in the form of a chart, with a copy for my family doctor. I was surprised to find that I came in the risk area for fractures.

After a chat about diet, supplements and exercise, they gave me a booklet which, among other information, showed the calcium content of a range of foods. The half-hour had been a pleasant experience, all the more so because it was not in a hospital setting, and it provided the information and the motivation for me to take better care of my bones. Incidentally, ultrasound has two important features:

1 It does not involve any radiation – important if you could be pregnant.
2 The information from a heel examination tells if you are at risk of a hip fracture, but is not as informative about your spine.

Bone density

It is useful to know your bone mass or BMD even before you have reached the age and hormonal stage when bone loss is definitely outstripping bone replacement, since then you have a base-line measurement for assessing your progress later. Some of us lose bone slowly at the change, while in others it is so rapid that treatment is urgently required, with further checks to monitor how well it is working.

What should send you for an examination of your bone density now
You have no symptoms and you feel OK, but:

For a woman:
- Episodes in the past when your periods stopped for several months.
- Irregular periods always.
- Periods started late – 15 or older.
- Menopause came early – 45 or less.
- You have had anorexia nervosa, although you are now fully recovered.
- Excessive physical exercise while training.
- Gynaecological operations, especially involving the ovaries.
- Chemotherapy for cancer anywhere.
- Radiotherapy in the pelvic region.

For either sex:
- Developmental problems involving the sexual organs.
- Any previous fracture.
- Bones breaking easily.
- Chronic over-use of alcohol.
- Hooked on cigarettes.
- Sedentary lifestyle.
- Long period of immobilization after injury or illness.
- Longstanding disease – for example, overactive thyroid, Cushing's disease, chronic kidney disorder, haemophilia, insulin-dependent diabetes, multiple sclerosis.
- Taking steroids or anticonvulsants long term.
- Prolonged heparin infusion for clotting problem.
- Incidental discovery of osteopenia – transparent bones in an X-ray, although no fracture.

Alex

Alex was upset because, at 55, he could not perform sexually and, to tell the truth, he had lost the feeling for it. His wife, who was a few years older than him, was not worried by the lack of marital relations. They had been declining over several years.

A physical examination showed nothing wrong with Alex's sexual organs, but he was overweight with a beer belly and slight breast swellings. Liver function tests showed some damage, and he had a low testosterone level. He was suffering from hypogonadism – underproduction of the sex hormones. Their natural slow decline had been speeded up by the effect of too much alcohol. The lack of sex hormones put him in line for osteoporosis, even more than a menopausal woman. It was important to check the state of his bones since he could well be at a high risk of fracture.

His firm paid for their employees' medical insurance so Alex was able to have a DEXA test straight away. This involved nothing more arduous than lying still while the X-ray machine rolled above him, taking pictures of his whole body. It took about ten minutes. The results showed that he was well into osteoporosis. His treatment included a testosterone implant, equivalent to HRT for a woman.

Diagnosing osteoporosis

In times past, the diagnosis of osteoporosis was made with the naked eye. The characteristic picture was of a short, thin woman, severely stooped and with a dowager's hump. This was one form of hunchback – a horrible term that went out a hundred years ago.

DIY instant check for bone loss

Get someone to measure your arm span, from fingertip to fingertip, horizontally. If this is more than your height it is likely that your vertebrae are giving way because the bone is getting weaker, due to osteoporosis, and becoming compressed. A small part of the loss of height is due to the shrinkage of the discs of gristle between the bones.

Low bone mass and low mineral density

Low bone mass and low mineral density always go together. They are the tell-tale signs of osteoporosis and predict the likelihood of a fracture and all that may entail. Low scores also crop up in osteopenia and osteomalacia, but these are basically stages in the development of osteoporosis (see p. 7).

The tests

Several techniques for measuring bone mass and BMD have been developed over the last half-century, but particularly in the last decade. All of them depend on complex technology, and their accuracy is of vital importance since the smallest changes in bone mass or density reflect very big changes in bone strength.

X-rays

Simple X-rays show reduced density by increased transparency of the bones, especially those in the wrist and hand. An X-ray taken when there has been a fracture, or perhaps for a chest problem, is often how the diagnosis of osteoporosis is first made. Sadly, by the time it can be detected on film, 40 per cent of the bone's mineral strength has been lost.

Radiogrammetry

Radiogrammetry compares the whole width of a bone with the width of its hard, outer cortex and hence the width of the trabecular or cancellous inner part. The osteoporotic process affects this type of bone first and most severely, but the mineral content of the bone is found mainly in the cortex. It is evidence of a substantial loss of solid bone if the total width of the cortical part is less than that of the trabecular bone. This method of assessing osteoporosis is approximate, at best, and only works for bones of a convenient long shape. It is not applicable to the severest cases, since in these the cortical bone has become porous, like the cancellous type.

Qualitative spinal morphometry

This impressive-sounding mouthful describes another method of assessing bone density from X-rays. It has been in use for over 50 years and amounts to a system of grading based on the arrangement of the bone scaffolding in the trabecular bone. As more and more bone is lost it is the horizontal trabeculae which are eliminated, leaving a pattern of vertical stripes.

The Singh Index

This is a similar ploy, but based on the arrangement of the trabeculae in a triangle of bone – Ward's triangle – at the upper end of the thigh bone. The index comprises six classes, but unfortunately they do not accord well with BMD values obtained by the newer DEXA technique. Both of these morphometric methods rely rather heavily on subjective judgements.

DEXA: dual energy X-ray absorptiometry

DEXA is the 'gold standard' technique for assessing bone density. The principle depends on the reduction in numbers and intensity of the photons emitted by the X-rays as they pass through the bone and other tissues. Dense – or solid – material attenuates the photons more than that of a looser structure, and it is the degree of attenuation that is measured. The DEXA machine is set to differentiate bone from soft tissue and to assess the solidity of the bones. A built-in computer converts this into numbers and the BMD of the bones in different areas can be read off directly.

DEXA can be used for any bone in the body and is less affected than other forms of X-ray by the amount of fat in the vicinity. However, osteoarthritis of the lower – lumbar – region of the spine, and calcification of the aorta, the main artery leaving the heart, can interfere with the results. To get round this, a lateral view as well as the front-to-back view can be taken. This involves exposure to more radiation, but the dose is very small – it is only likely to be relevant in the case of early pregnancy. The image from the side enhances the differences between normal and osteoporotic bone.

Fractures of the vertebrae appear as denser areas of bone since the bone is compressed as it partially collapses.

Tessa

Tessa had excessively heavy periods, especially since her third baby, and she and her doctor finally decided that she should have a hysterectomy, but to leave the ovaries untouched so as to avoid severe hot flushes and other menopausal symptoms. She was 38, far too young to think about osteoporosis in the ordinary way, but her doctor wanted to know the state of her bones at the time of the operation, as a basis for monitoring any changes that might take place in reaction to the hysterectomy.

He arranged a DEXA examination. Tessa did not need to undress, but as usual with X-rays she had to take her jewellery off. All she had to do was to lie still on the machine, basically a long box, while the X-ray arm moved slowly along the length of her body about 18 inches above her. The whole process took less than 15 minutes and she felt nothing.

Tessa's BMD for hips and spine was near the average for her age and sex, but she is to have a re-run in six months to check for changes.

QCT: quantitative computerized tomography

QCT is an advance on the old CAT or CT scan, but similarly provides a picture representing X-rays of a series of thin transverse slices through the body. These can be built up into a three-dimensional image. From this it is possible to work out the BMD of the bone in any part. The only snags are the high running cost of the apparatus and a higher dose of radiation than with other methods. To keep it in perspective, however, the amount of radiation from a QCT scan is about the same as that from a flight across the Atlantic.

Quantitative ultrasound

The technique of ultrasound is best known for its use in imaging unborn babies – a guarantee of its safety in this respect, compared with methods involving radiation. It works by sending inaudible – to us – sound waves through the area being investigated, and measuring how fast they travel (velocity of sound or VOS) and how quickly they lose their strength (attenuation) and what surfaces they bounce off, like echoes. The process takes five minutes, gives an instant answer in bone units on a chart and is completely safe and painless (see p. 43). Its disadvantage is that while it works well, using the cancellous bone of the heel, for assessing the bone mass of the hip region, particularly in women of 70-plus, it is not as useful for examining the spine.

The usefulness of knowing your BMD and bone mass

- Finding out if you have osteoporosis.
- Monitoring your progress over years.

- Assessing the need for HRT.
- Checking the effect of steroids and other long-term medication.
- Assessing the dangers of a fracture – there is a baseline for any given age and sex and bone mass.

Many modern GPs have a bone scanner in their surgeries – usually ultrasound.

One proviso: people who are unduly thin or rather fat may have unreliable results from these methods of assessing bone mass and density. If you do not have much fat on your body your bone mass will seem to be higher, while if you are plump it will seem lower. As you get older you accumulate fat in your bone marrow and this can be enough to distort the values.

Laboratory tests

Laboratory tests provide background information about your general health and certain illnesses. Two disorders, in particular, may be deceptive – overactive thyroid, or thyrotoxicosis, and myeloma. Without tests either may go unrecognized, and yet cause osteoporosis. A simple blood test shows up any excess of thyroxine in the blood, which may be due to thyrotoxicosis or, just as likely, to over-generous prescribing of the hormone for those with underactive glands. Myeloma can be detected by a blood test showing anaemia and a urine test showing an undue loss of protein.

Biochemical tests in the assessment of osteoporosis

Established osteoporosis comes in two types which are probably the opposite ends of the spectrum.

1 *Active*, in which there is a fast rate of bone removal and renewal, with loss of bone minerals, mainly calcium.
2 *Inactive*, in which the turnover is slow. The small extra loss of calcium in the urine that occurs as resorption overtakes bone formation in the middle years is offset by the equally age-related decrease in the absorption of calcium from the intestine. The net result is little or no change in the level of calcium in the blood or urine.

It is important, when choosing the treatment, to identify the fast-track, active type since this is more dangerous. Luckily it also responds better to medication – with calcitonin in particular. In these cases it is urgent to rev up the other ploys and precautions against a fracture, too.

Biochemical tests come into their own when it comes to the assessment of the rate of bone turnover, resorption and formation.

Bone resorption is reflected in the urine. A big increase of calcium, hypercalciuria, occurs when bone is being broken down rapidly, as in active osteoporosis, and some other conditions. Other markers in the urine are *hydroxyproline* and *pyridinoline*. For a calcium estimation the urine must be collected throughout the 24 hours, but two hours suffices for either of the other two chemicals. While it is cheap and easy, although time-consuming, to measure the amount of calcium in the urine, it is not very helpful. Calcium levels are variable, day to day and even hour to hour, being influenced by what you eat, vitamin D, parathyroid hormone, salt intake and even the time of day.

Hydroxyproline or pyridinoline urine tests are standard for assessing how fast resorption is taking place.

One blood test, BGP, standing for bone Gla protein, confirms the urine tests. Bone proteins are released into the circulation as the bone is broken down. A high rate of bone turnover occurs in young, growing children, following a fracture, or in Paget's disease. The latter affects the bones of older people, particularly the shin bones and skull, which undergo a mix of very active bone formation and resorption, making for oversize, weak bones, warm to the touch through the skin. It is a kind of osteoporosis.

Bone formation accelerates too, as part of increased turnover. An increase in alkaline phosphatase in the serum is the chief marker for this. It is slightly raised in osteoporosis. Other causes are:

- recent fracture;
- anticonvulsants and some other drugs;
- secondary bone cancer.

Osteocalcin

Osteocalcin is a bone protein manufactured by the osteoblasts (bone-building cells). The amount in the serum is increased when there is rapid turnover with extra bone formation, but it only shows up sometimes in osteoporosis so it is unreliable as a test for the disorder.

All in all, the biochemical tests are a little disappointing for the detective work in osteoporosis, but improvements are in the pipeline. Anyway, the excellence of the tests like DEXA and quantitative ultrasound, based on physics, and the new technology more than compensate.

7

Treatment 1: Hormonal

It can come as a shock, or if you already have an inkling it strikes a chill, when you are told that you have osteoporosis. One thing you must not do is brush the information aside because you feel perfectly OK – you are not a geriatric, and you live a healthy lifestyle. Remember the sneakiness of osteoporosis, the way it creeps up on you and then, suddenly a bone breaks for hardly any reason, or your back starts playing up.

You should not underestimate the significance of the diagnosis, but do not let it depress you either. It is not as though there is nothing you – and your doctor – can do. There is plenty of DIY in the matter of diet and lifestyle, and a whole range of effective modern medicines to deal with the situation. It may not be possible to put back bone that has been lost, but your bones can certainly be strengthened by the treatment, setting up an insurance against future fractures.

The strands of treatment

1 Lifestyle and diet each merit a chapter of their own (see Chapters 13 and 14). They are bound up with prevention and will apply regardless of other therapy you may have. Take it as read that you must have enough calcium, vitamin D and exercise.
2 Calcium as treatment (see Chapter 8).
3 Medication geared especially for osteoporosis (see Chapter 9).
4 Hormone treatments, dealt with in this chapter.

HRT

The sex hormones, in women specifically oestrogen, maintain the strength of the bones. For men, read testosterone. These hormones work by moderating the rate of bone turnover and the consequent loss of minerals. Net bone loss from the resorption/formation cycle runs at less than 1 per cent of the total bone, per year, for both sexes until – for women only – the menopause disrupts the situation. The reduction in oestrogen production is sudden and substantial, with an immediate jump in the rate of bone loss to more than double: 2 to 3 per cent per year. For men any change is small and gradual.

The dramatic decrease in bone strength is reflected in the increase in the number of women of 45-plus who suffer from fractures after minimal trauma. Any bone will crack under whatever strain is too much for it, and this can be very little with a weakened bone. Fractures of the wrist, hip and spine are the commonest, and as well as immediate ill-effects, they all have some that are longer term. Having had one fracture makes you more likely to have another – unless you take HRT, hormone replacement therapy. This is basically oestrogen with or without progestogen.

Contraindications

Not everyone can safely take HRT.

Absolute no-nos

- Cancer of the breast or womb.
- Pregnancy.
- Undiagnosed bleeding from the vagina.
- Melanoma.
- Serious liver disease.

Relative contraindications

- Very high blood pressure.
- Migraine.
- Gallstones.
- Diabetes.
- Mild liver disease.
- Previous breast or uterine cancer.
- Previous deep vein thrombosis (DVT) or embolism.
- Endometriosis.
- Fibroids.

In these cases extra care and frequent check-ups are needed. If major surgery is planned there should be a six-week gap without the medication before and after the operation.

Warnings and side-effects

If you are taking HRT stop at once if you have any of the following symptoms, or if you think you are pregnant:

- migraine-type headaches (one-sided, with nausea and disturbed vision) occurring for the first time;
- frequent severe headaches of any type;
- sudden visual disturbance;
- rise in blood pressure since starting HRT;
- jaundice.

Side-effects which are troublesome, but not dangerous, include:

- stomach upset;
- nausea, vomiting;
- tenderness of the breasts;
- putting on weight;
- mild headaches, dizziness;
- nosebleeds;
- itchy skin.

Erica

Erica was 52 when she slipped and fell against a table and broke two ribs. They healed quickly, but at this time she began having twinges of severe pain in her lower back. Physiotherapy did not help much, and an X-ray showed her bones were more transparent than normal, so the doctor arranged a DEXA bone scan for Erica. It revealed unmistakable osteoporosis.

A snag was that Erica had quite a large fibroid. It was causing no trouble and Erica certainly did not want an operation. She was started on a sequential oestrogen/progestogen tablet – the progestogen was given during the last part of the cycle. All went well to start with, but then Erica had an exceptionally heavy 'period' and the following month the bleed was not only heavy but painful. HRT was not for Erica unless she had a hysterectomy. She did not want to lose her womb, but the fibroid was too large and awkward to be removed on its own. Instead, Erica is taking etidronate, one of the bisphosphonate medicines, and doing well (see p. 68).

New views on HRT

Until two or three years ago, HRT was considered to be the answer to all the problems of middle-aged women, including osteoporosis, heart disease and stroke as well as menopausal symptoms. Since then, breast cancer has been on the increase, up 5.1 per cent during the year 2000–2001. It is now the second most common cause of death from cancer in women, and the main cause of death among women in the 40–55 age group.

It is strongly suspected, though not proven, that the oestrogen component of HRT is a major cause of the disease.

HRT is no longer considered to be one of the best treatments for osteoporosis since the advent of the bisphosphonates (see Chapter 9), and even more recently Forsteo (teriparatide) and Protelos (strontium ranelate) (see p. 73). HRT is no longer recommended as a preventative of heart disease or stroke, but is still the most effective treatment for menopausal symptoms.

Anorexia nervosa

The obsessive starvation illness, which affects teenage girls most frequently, prevents the building of a good bone mass in the long term. In severe cases it can lead to teenage osteoporosis, demonstrated by the occurrence of unexpected fractures, and confirmed by BMD assessment. Some experts have considered that HRT would be helpful in these cases and have had some success, while others have tried it with poor results. In fact the hormone is irrelevant compared with the urgent need to restore the girl's weight – when she will be able to make her own oestrogen from the natural fat, cholesterol.

Men

Men are far less liable than women to a sharp, substantial fall in sex hormone production. This is reflected in their much smaller likelihood of an osteoporotic fracture. The lifetime risk of hip fracture for a (white) woman is 15 per cent; for a man it is 5 per cent. The lifetime risk of a wrist fracture for a woman is 15 per cent; for a man it is 2 per cent.

Bone loss for men runs at 0.3 per cent per year, only increasing slightly in old age, while for women it shoots up to 2.2 to 3 per cent around the menopause. However, men are not immune from a shortage of sex hormones and the testosterone level has been shown to correlate negatively with BMD, at least in the hip area. Hypogonadism can occur developmentally, and after delayed puberty. Heavy smoking (three or more packs a day) or alcohol in excess can cause it, with marked loss of bone, and steroid medication long term has an even stronger deleterious effect. Finally, while most men show only a mild decline, in some men their sex hormone output is reduced drastically in middle age – for no obvious reason. This is called *idiopathic* osteoporosis – doctor-speak for 'we don't understand it'. Apart from hormone deficit, in men past 50, as with women, the absorption of calcium from the intestine is less efficient, and they need to keep up their supplies of calcium and vitamin D in the senior years when they are bound to have some degree of osteoporosis.

Testosterone

Testosterone, the male equivalent of oestrogen, can be used in treatment but it is not so simple to take. Tablets do not work, leaving these choices:

- injections two to four times weekly;
- patches, applied to the scrotum;
- an implant.

The big disadvantage of testosterone treatment is that it tends to cause enlargement of the prostate gland – already a problem in many men from middle age onwards. Other possible side-effects are an increased, perhaps undue interest in sex, and aggression.

Delayed puberty in men, which is associated with hypogonadism, can be treated with testosterone injections but usually does better with an anabolic steroid, such as nandrolone.

SERMS

Raloxifene (Evista) is one of a class of drugs known as Selective (O)Estrogen Receptor Modulators (SERMs). This is a synthetic drug which mimics oestrogen in working against osteoporosis, especially of the spine, reducing cholesterol and countering heart and artery disease. At the same time it functions as an anti-oestrogen in its action on the breast and womb where it reduces the risk of cancer – a winner all round.

Raloxifene is specifically recommended and licensed for women past the menopause who have a low BMD in their vertebrae, with a high chance of deformity and back pain. You only need to take one tablet a day.

Contraindications

Do not take raloxifene if you have:
- severe liver disease;
- severe kidney disease;
- cancer of the breast or womb;
- unexplained bleeding from the vagina;
- previous blood clots;
- a chronic disorder with the likelihood of being laid up for a long time.

Precautions

- Be sure to have plenty of calcium while you are on this medicine.
- Check that you are not taking any medicine containing oestrogen (except ointments) or cholestyramine (Questran).

Beneficial effects

- Improvement in BMD.
- Reduction of 50 per cent in fracture risk in the back, hip and other bones.
- Reduced risk of heart attack.

Possible side-effects

You are very likely to have none, but they may include:
- hot flushes or other menopausal symptoms;
- leg cramps;
- swollen ankles;
- blood clots – risk similar to HRT.

Claire

Claire was 55, three years past her last period, and not keen to have any more of such bothers. Her family medical history included her father who had angina, an uncle who died of a coronary, and an aunt and one grandmother who had suffered from breast cancer. Her doctor felt she should not have HRT because of this history, but she needed to avoid osteoporosis. Regular mammograms showed that Claire had perfectly normal breasts, and the only other feature of interest was her blood pressure – borderline raised at 150/88. She had read about raloxifene and was keen to try it, but the specialist would not prescribe it. Although theoretically it would have been ideal for Claire's situation, there was not yet enough evidence to feel totally confident in using it for people with breast cancer in their family.

Claire, with her doctor, settled for one of the bisphosphonate medicines when a bone density scan showed that she was in the risk area for a fracture. She has not had any bone trouble to date.

Calcitonin

This hormone was discovered in 1961 and 30 years later was introduced into the treatment of osteoporosis. It is produced by the thyroid gland, together with the two thyroid hormones, but instead of being under central command calcitonin is controlled through the amount of calcium in the circulation. A high level of calcium links in with increased release of calcitonin, and vice versa. This hormone prevents resorption by disabling the osteoclasts. In this it has the opposite effect to parathyroid hormone which stimulates the breakdown of bone.

If you have a lot of calcium in your diet – cheese, milk, yogurt, greens – this leads to a cutback in parathyroid hormone and an increase in bone-saving calcitonin, especially in men. Women, in fact, may spend their whole lives producing barely enough calcitonin to protect their bones from the osteoclasts. Blood tests show that post-menopausal women with osteoporosis have a much reduced output of this valuable hormone and a reduced reserve.

Treatment with calcitonin

Its first use was not for osteoporosis, but in:

- Paget's disease of bone;
- hypercalcaemia (excess calcium in the blood) from any cause, e.g. thyrotoxicosis, various cancers, especially myeloma, overactive parathyroids;
- vitamin D toxicity in cases of excessive dosage;
- immobilization, long term, as in paraplegics;
- steroid medicines, long term.

In 1989 calcitonin was finally recognized as a useful treatment in osteoporosis. The effects of calcitonin therapy in osteoporosis are:

- less breakdown of bone;
- less loss of bone;
- increased bone mass;
- remodelling, over time, of deformed bones;
- improved quality of bone as assessed by ultrasound, raised BMD;
- less risk of a trapped nerve in the spine.

Calcitonin is especially effective in active osteoporosis with rapid bone loss, so it is useful, before deciding on treatment, to find out which type you have (see p. 19). Active osteoporosis is flagged up by:

- urine tests for hydroxyproline or pyridinoline;
- blood test for BGP, bone Gla protein.

Painkilling effect

The acute pain of crushed and fractured vertebrae is relieved by calcitonin in 75 per cent of cases, by the natural method of stimulating the production of the body's own painkillers, the endorphins. It is of some help in chronic back pain if it is due to osteoporosis.

The main uses of calcitonin today

- Osteoporosis in post-menopausal women for whom HRT is contraindicated or who are anxious because of a family or personal history of cancer of the breast or womb. This also applies to those with an overactive thyroid or on steroid therapy.
- As a preventive for athletes who are putting their bones at risk by a great deal of exercise and do not want the fattening effect of HRT.
- After oophorectomy – removal of the ovaries – it is as effective as oestrogen in this situation of oestrogen deficiency.

Taking calcitonin

It is usually taken as salcatonin (Calsynar, Miacalcic). This is a synthetic form of salmon calcitonin which has a stronger effect than the human variety. The big snag is that it cannot be taken by mouth. That leaves two possibilities:

1 Injection, preferably subcutaneous – that is, just under the skin rather than into the muscle. You need a dose five times a week for bone pain, three to five times for osteoporosis without pain. Most people soon learn to give themselves the injections.
2 Nasal spray must be used daily; it is just as efficacious as the injection, but with a smaller total dosage.

Whichever route is used, improvements in BMD, especially in the back, begin to show in six to eight months, with a measurable reduction in fracture risk after 18 to 24 months. Sometimes the beneficial response to the treatment plateaus at this stage, and some specialists then change to a system of treatment in alternate years, in the hope of achieving the best long-term effect. Pain due to a crush fracture is reduced in the early part of treatment and does not usually return unless there is a new lesion. The mending of the broken bone is quicker with this treatment.

Side-effects

In general, these are less likely with the spray than with the injections, and less likely with subcutaneous than with intramuscular jabs. None of these side-effects is likely to persist.

- Aching or pain at the injection site – in 10 per cent.
- Irritation in the nose – in 12 per cent.
- Flushing of the face – in 8 to 10 per cent.
- Nausea – in less than 3 per cent: it can be prevented by taking the medicine at bedtime, with an anti-emetic.
- Very occasionally there is vomiting and diarrhoea.

Helen

Helen was 84, thin but spry. She had lived on her own and coped with her own very limited cooking and cleaning and self-care. One of the hardest jobs was the shopping. Her health had been good and the only operation she had had was a hysterectomy for heavy losses when she was 44. At that time HRT was not in general use and her doctor had not suggested it.

She had been having niggling pains in the lumbar region and her left knee was mildly arthritic. On one shopping trip, when the pavements were wet, she slipped but managed to save herself by grabbing a stand outside the newsagents. It was after this that she had really troublesome pains in her back. Her doctor said she had low back pain syndrome and explained that quite a lot of elderly ladies had pure osteopenia, a thinning of the bone without the breakdown of its structure that means osteoporosis. Osteopenia alone does not cause pain. Or she might have arthritis in her back as well as her knee, and that could be the cause of her pain. An X-ray showed arthritis, but also the flattened shape of crushed osteoporotic vertebrae, with one distinctly wedge-shaped, presumably from a specific bending injury. For arthritis the usual prescription is one of the non-steroidal anti-inflammatory drugs (NSAIDs) such as ibuprofen, if paracetamol is not effective, but Helen had clear osteoporosis with indications that she damaged a bone when she nearly fell. The smallest injury is enough to break osteoporotic bone.

She did not want to start HRT at her age and was worried by what she had heard about fluoride, so she decided to brave the injections with calcitonin, and to take all the advice on avoiding falls (see p. 91). Six months later her back pain has nearly gone, and she is trying without the medication – apart from supplements of calcium and vitamin D.

Other hormones

Tamoxifen

This is an anti-oestrogen used in breast cancer and when there is a high risk of it, to counter the influence of oestrogen. It has contradictory effects on bone – not all bad, as would have been expected. If you have passed the menopausal stage and therefore are not producing much oestrogen, tamoxifen has a protective effect on your bones, but we do not know what its effect may be on younger women with plenty of oestrogen. Tamoxifen may be useful in some post-menopausal women who cannot take oestrogen. The main side-effects are hot flushes, headache, digestive and liver upsets, eye problems, bleeding from the vagina and an increased risk of clotting. The last three are a warning to stop the medication.

Progesterone

This is a progestogen, sometimes used without oestrogen as a contraceptive. It has a deleterious effect on the bone mass, and the depot preparations are particularly harmful, especially in young women who should still be building up their bone reserves. Medroxyprogesterone acetate, MPA, is an exception: it does not interfere with the beneficial effects of oestrogen, and itself prevents hot flushes and sweats. Some other progestogens have an anabolic effect – that is, tissue-building – but are not used in osteoporosis.

Growth hormone

As you would expect, the production of this hormone hits a high during the growth spurt of adolescence and declines as you get older. It has been suggested that lack of growth hormone underlies the deterioration in the strength of the skeleton over time. It is in particularly short supply in elderly men with idiopathic (unexplained) osteoporosis. A six-month course of injections leads to an increase in muscle, fat, skin thickness, and bone density, especially in the back. It is only suitable for senior men.

Anabolic steroids

Stanozolol and nandrolone are those in common use. They lead to an increase in muscle and a decrease in fat, with improved mobility and confidence – the reasons for their use by athletes. They increase the total body calcium and BMD in the vertebrae, and reduce the number of fractures – and over three years are more effective than HRT. They are given by monthly injection.

Since they are derivatives of testosterone it is understandable that they may have an effect on facial hair and the depth of the voice and it is these side-effects which cause 30 per cent of women to give them up, despite their beneficial effect on osteoporosis, especially back pain. The virilizing effects are no drawback for older men. Other possible side-effects include acne, increased libido, fluid retention and liver problems, including the tumour, hepatoma.

Other drugs

Fluoride

Minute amounts, one part per million in the water supply, have been shown to strengthen the teeth against decay. There also seemed to be fewer fractures of the vertebrae in areas where the water was fluoridated. For this reason it has been used as a treatment in osteoporosis.

On the plus side it certainly stimulates bone formation, but there are doubts about the structure of the trabecular bone produced – the type most susceptible to fracture in osteoporosis. However, 30 to 60 per cent of those with osteoporosis who take fluoride long term show an improvement in bone density as demonstrated by X-ray, and after five years this may even reach normal values. A mix of fluoride, calcium and vitamin D, taken for three months or more improves backache due to osteoporosis – but there are other causes for this common complaint.

One of the disadvantages that have damped the enthusiasm for fluoride treatment is the statistic that while vertebral fractures decrease, the risk for wrist and hip and other fractures actually increases and after one vertebral fracture there is no reduction in the risk of recurrence. In general fluoride gives some protection against crush fractures, but not against twisting or bending. Another difficulty is working out the most effective dosage. While small to moderate doses boost bone strength, large doses reduce it.

Then of course there are the side-effects: these are worse if the fluoride is taken in a liquid than as tablets. They crop up often, but do not usually continue for long, and include:

- irritation of the digestive system: nausea, vomiting, pain and diarrhoea;
- bleeding from the digestive tract, severe enough to cause anaemia;
- bone pain;
- joint pain;
- kidney damage – rarely.

Although fluoride is not yet fully approved officially as a treatment for osteoporosis, work is in progress on making a slow-release preparation.

Thiazide diuretics

Thiazide water tablets are a cheap, effective treatment for high blood pressure. They also have the additional benefit – for those with osteoporosis – of decreasing the amount of calcium lost to the body in the urine. This leads to an increase in bone density, demonstrated in studies on the wrist and heel in elderly people. In those who have used thiazide for six years or more there is a 30 per cent reduction in the risk of a hip fracture.

One of the disadvantages of thiazides is that they reduce the amount of vitamin D in circulation and the amount of calcium absorbed from the intestine, and may leave the body depleted of magnesium, which can upset the rhythm of the heart.

Samson

Samson had hypercalciuria – too much calcium in his urine – due to the direct effect of an excess of thyroid hormone. He was well on the way to osteoporosis at 55. As well as an overactive thyroid, and linked with it, he had high blood pressure – 160/99 without treatment. His doctor prescribed carbimazole tablets to control his overactive thyroid, and for his high blood pressure, bendrofluazide, a thiazide diuretic. The latter, he felt, would counteract too much loss of calcium when there was no longer an excess of thyroid hormone, and protect his bone mineral strength. Samson was warned about the interaction with alcohol. The medic knew that he was not taking any of the incompatible drugs such as lithium, barbiturates or anti-inflammatories.

When Samson had been on the medication for six months he had a bone densitometry test and a thyroxine estimation. The thyroxine level was, if anything, a little below normal and his BMD result put him just clear of the risk level for osteoporotic fractures. His progress will be monitored every few months in case his medication needs adjustment.

8

Treatment 2: Calcium

Calcium is the first-line treatment for osteoporosis. Everyone knows that an adequate supply of calcium is a must for healthy bones, and that most of it – 75 per cent – comes from dairy products. Milk – full-cream, semi-skimmed or skimmed – and cheese are the richest sources, except for cottage cheese, which lags behind, for all its reputation for being 'good for you'.

A sad truth is that we in the West have been reducing our intake of these valuable foods over the last 40 years, partly through our fear of cholesterol, and partly due to our efforts to lose weight. The latter applies particularly to adolescent girls who are constantly slimming. A one-calorie Coke is cool, while a milk shake is not. A majority of teenage girls are taking less than their minimum requirement of calcium, never thinking that they are flirting with osteoporosis, later if not now. Those who run into true anorexia nervosa may also give themselves teenagers' osteoporosis with unexpected fractures.

Supplements of calcium, with its partner vitamin D, are essential treatment for these youngsters and any others whose diets provide too little of these items to maintain the strength of their skeletons – despite the abundance of food all round. The varying requirement for calcium is linked to the time of life.

Birth to early adulthood

Babies and the very young have a milk-based diet and all the calcium they need. Adolescents lay down 60 per cent of their adult bone mass during two or three vital years between the ages of 12 and 16 (girls) and 14 to 18 (boys). By 18, girls have 95 per cent of their peak bone mass, but with plenty of calcium may add to it slowly for another ten years. Males build up their bone mass steadily until they are about 30, with no setbacks like slimming, pregnancy or breastfeeding. They also benefit their bones by taking more exercise than girls, in general. Their peak bone mass, the insurance policy against osteoporosis later, is substantially higher than for females.

During the bone-growing adolescent period, calcium, covered by vitamin D, is the essential building material. It also preserves bone minerals by slowing down the rate of bone turnover. Supplements may well be beneficial during adolescence, and have been shown to lead to a higher peak bone mass in ordinary, normal youngsters.

Later requirements for calcium

The body has its own automatic mechanism for correcting a shortage of calcium. It reacts by increasing the output of parathyroid hormone. This in turn increases the amount of calcium absorbed from the gut, and also increases the amount saved by the kidneys from being passed out in the urine.

This system works well between the ages of 25 and 45, when there are no longer the extra demands of adolescence, but before the drastic fall-off in oestrogen of the menopause. From 45 onwards, in the run-up to the change, the ovaries gradually give up the business of releasing eggs and making sex hormones. Bone turnover accelerates and there is a sharp loss of calcium. Men up to age 65 and women before the menopause lose about 20 g of calcium daily, which is comfortably replaced from their diet. With the menopause the loss escalates to 60 g daily, but you do not suddenly take three times as much calcium in your food. This high rate of loss continues for six or seven years before settling – this is the time to take a calcium supplement.

The perimenopausal period

At this time around the menopause, most women are teetering on the edge of osteoporosis. Some of them succumb, and fractures from surprisingly minor trauma begin to crop up. You may not realize what is happening to you and your bones. This is a good time to check, as best you can, how much calcium you are getting from your diet. You need 1000 mg daily if you are on HRT or 1500 mg otherwise. Extra calcium will help to keep up your bone density at this age but the greatest need is for oestrogen, especially phyto-oestrogens.

About five years after your menopause your rate of bone – and calcium – loss becomes less alarmingly rapid and settles to a steady, continuous leakage with men and women on an equal footing. However, bone loss never comes to a complete halt. The neat compensatory arrangement that saved calcium in your middle adult years no longer works as you get older. This is partly due to failure of absorption and partly because the kidneys become less efficient at conserving calcium.

The Third Age

Those in their seventies and eighties, and even more senior, need more calcium and vitamin D than they can get from their food. Calcium supplementation definitely helps them. And no one is too old to benefit. In one study, osteoporosis sufferers of average age 84 were given a daily dose of 1000 mg of calcium and 800 mg of vitamin D, then closely monitored. After six months their bones showed some improvement and after 18 months there was a reduction in all types of fracture apart from those of the vertebrae, but including a 30 per cent less risk of hip fracture. There was also an overall drop in deaths, compared with those not taking the medication (they were too old to have a great expectation of life).

Calcium worked more quickly in cutting the risk of fracture than any of the pharmaceutical medicines.

How to take calcium

There is a wide choice of preparations.

- Tablets of various calcium salts, mostly with added vitamin D. Calcium carbonate (chalk) is most commonly used, but calcium citrate is particularly useful for people with a lack of stomach acid.
- Chewable tablets – for example, Calcichew.
- Calcidrink.
- Calcium in syrup.
- Calcium in a carton of orange juice.

Contraindications

Do not take calcium if tests have shown that you have:

- hypercalcaemia (too much calcium in your blood);
- hypercalciuria (too much calcium in your urine);
- kidney stones;
- sarcoidosis.

Diabetes

Take special care if you have diabetes, checking your blood sugar meticulously. If you are taking other medicines for osteoporosis, find out whether you should be taking them at a separate time from the calcium.

Interactions

Calcium may interact with:

- tetracycline;
- thiazide water tablets (see p. 60);
- fluoride supplements (see p. 59);
- steroids;
- barbiturates;
- iron;
- digoxin.

It may also interact with high doses of vitamin D, and bisphosphonates: important anti-osteoporosis medicines (see p. 67).

Side-effects

Usually there are none, but the possibilities include:

- stomach upset, indigestion;
- constipation;
- bloating, wind.

For maximum efficacy calcium is best taken at bedtime. In the night there is an increase in bone turnover and an extra loss of calcium in the urine – unless you take a supplement in the late evening.

Hydroxyapatite (Ossopan)

This medicine is derived directly from bone and provides calcium and phosphate. It comes in sachets and should be taken twice a day before meals, the second time in the late evening.

The only contraindications are hypercalcaemia and hypercalciuria, but there should be careful monitoring in the case of kidney stones or serious kidney disorder. No side-effects are described.

Kirsty

Kirsty was green, feminist and a romantic. She bought her food in a health store and was practically a vegan as a matter of principle. She cut out dairy products and eggs among other nutrients. She was tall and very thin – willowy when she was younger, but gaunt at 53.

She and her friend, who held similar views, liked to be close to nature and went on walking holidays, covering miles and miles and feeling smug and healthy. Kirsty could hardly believe it when she was told that she had two broken ribs. She had felt a sharp pain in her chest during a fit of laughing – and it did not pass off. At the hospital they found localized spots of pain and tenderness on her ribs, and the lateral X-ray showed that several of her vertebrae were crumbling, although her back had not hurt until now. The diagnosis was moderately severe osteoporosis – the disease would not have shown up on an ordinary X-ray without there being a loss of 35 to 40 per cent of the bone substance.

Although her periods had stopped about three years earlier, Kirsty had not had HRT because she felt it was 'unnatural' and she was not willing to take it now. She also refused the doctor's next suggestion – alendronate (a bisphosphonate). Kirsty did not believe in straight medicine, so she fixed herself up with some aromatherapy, then the Alexander technique. They were both enjoyable but the back pain which had started when she broke her ribs got worse. Her mother of 84 argued fiercely with Kirsty and got her to agree to take calcium and vitamin D from the health food shop. She also took a complex of the B vitamins which she lacked on her limited diet. She had a little trouble with constipation, which was unusual for her: this was probably due to a mild excess of calcium.

Kirsty's back pain lessened slightly over the months, but on such a low diet bone healing would be a protracted affair.

Your calcium needs

The list below suggests more calcium than the RDA (recommended daily dose) put out by the Department of Health, but accords with that of the National Osteoporosis Society in the UK and National Osteoporosis Foundation in the USA. You may get all you need from what you eat: see p. 111 for a list of food values. Dairy products are tops – $\frac{1}{3}$ pint (190 ml) of semi-skimmed milk provides 231 mg of calcium. The average calcium intake in both countries is just 870 mg, which falls far short of the needs of your body and bones.

To make use of the calcium you also need vitamin D – 400–800 i.u. daily until you hit retirement age, when it should be 800 i.u. The vitamin is less well absorbed as you get older, and you do not make as much through your skin. Fifteen to 20 minutes outside in the sunlight every day during the summer months will allow you to build a store that will last you all winter from childhood until 65. From then on, and particularly if you are confined to an indoor life in a nursing home or somewhere similar, you will need supplements by mouth. Fish liver oils – cod or halibut – as liquid or in capsules are an easy, effective way to make up the shortfall.

Recommended daily calcium intake

Under-fives	400–600 mg
Children up to age 11	800 mg
Teenagers	1000 mg
Men aged 20 to 60	1000 mg
Women aged 20 to 45	1000 mg
Pregnant and nursing women	1200 mg
Pregnant and nursing teenage mothers	1500 mg
Women over 45 without HRT	1500 mg
Women over 45 on HRT	1000 mg
Men aged over 60	1500 mg

Side-effects are more likely if you are taking more than 2000 mg daily, and especially if you are a senior.

9

Treatment 3: Bisphosphonates and recent advances – teriparatide

Bisphosphonates are man-made compounds which have been used for many years on the industrial scene for descaling pipes and boilers because of their capacity for preventing deposits of calcium carbonate – chalk. It was not until the late 1960s that they were first introduced into medicine. Their arrival has revolutionized the treatment of osteoporosis.

Because of their special affinity for calcium, bisphosphonates are attracted to bone. In particular, they concentrate on the surface of active, living bone, making it unappetizing for the osteoclasts whose function is to eat it away. Some of the dose of bisphosphonate is taken up by the bone cells and can remain embedded in the bone tissue for years.

Bisphosphonates were originally used to treat two conditions:

- Paget's disease, in which there is excessive bone activity with a high turnover and redundant bone formation.
- Hypercalcaemia, an excess of calcium in the blood often associated with some forms of cancer.

Bisphosphonates remain the top treatment for these conditions today, but in the early 1970s they were tried out on the modern plague of osteoporosis, with encouraging results. By the mid-1980s a wave of research studies was being carried out on their action and effectiveness in this disease – and they still continue. New drugs of the bisphosphonate class are constantly being developed and assessed in clinical trials against placebos and each other. The outlook is progressively more hopeful with each improvement.

A minor nuisance is that everything happens so slowly in bone disease, including osteoporosis, that every study takes years before it produces an answer.

The disorders which have been found to benefit from bisphosphonate treatment are:

- hypercalcaemia due to malignant disease;
- Paget's disease;
- metastatic bone disease, that is, secondaries in the bones from cancer of the breast, prostate, womb, etc.;
- multiple myeloma;

- immobilization, from whatever cause;
- rheumatoid arthritis;
- overactive parathyroid glands;
- osteogenesis imperfecta and other genetic disorders;
- bladder and kidney stones;
- osteoporosis – all types: juvenile, post-menopausal, senile, idiopathic, and steroid-induced.

While the effect of a bisphosphonate on hypercalcaemia is noticeable within hours of taking a dose, in Paget's disease and osteoporosis, due to the snail's-pace metabolism of bone, it takes months for the results to show. The manufacturers of alendronate (Fosamax) say that their drug causes a measurable increase in bone density within three months and a reduction in the risk of fracture within a year.

How bisphosphonates work

They have three actions relevant to osteoporosis:

1 Reduction in the rate of bone turnover. This in itself saves bone, particularly from the time of the menopause, when turnover increases dramatically, or after a fracture when there is a temporary flare-up.
2 Interference with the bone-destroying action, resorption, of the osteoclasts. After an initial boost to the number of cells, the effect of the drug is to prevent the half-formed osteoclasts from maturing. This means fewer active osteoclasts, and the result of this shows in the absence of the tiny pits on the surface of the bones where resorption has taken place.
3 A mixed effect on bone mineral density. In high dosage all the bisphosphonates inhibit the mineralization of bone, that is, the incorporation of calcium, giving them their strength. One of the earliest of the bisphosphonates, still in use, etidronate (Didronel) has this action even at a dosage commonly used in treatment. It can bring on osteomalacia or rickets from lack of calcium in the bones. With the other bisphosphonates, for instance the popular alendronate (Fosamax), this undesirable effect does not occur. Etidronate can only safely be given in low doses, and the BMD needs monitoring.

Taking bisphosphonates

These drugs are all poorly absorbed from the intestine when taken by mouth, which is obviously the most convenient way. To get the most out of your daily dose it is vital to take it when your stomach is completely empty, for instance when you wake up in the morning, before you have anything to eat or drink – no morning tea! You down the tablet with a full glass of tap water – no fancy mineral waters – and have nothing else to drink or eat for a full hour. Even then, you will only absorb between 1 and 5 per cent of the bisphosphonate. This is something to do with its having a negative charge which inhibits its diffusion through the membrane lining of the small intestine, the place where absorption, such as it is, occurs.

Any food in the stomach or intestine, especially if it contains calcium, reduces the absorption still more because it 'binds' the bisphosphonate into an insoluble form. Calcium supplements are even more potent. Half the medicine, after reaching your bloodstream, is completely cleared from it within 12 hours. It is passed out, unaltered, in your water. The other half is taken up by your bone cells and embedded in your skeleton. There it is apparently inert and is only very slowly removed over the years. In the case of alendronate (Fosamax), it takes ten years before half of the original amount in your skeleton has disappeared. It is the medicine in your blood and on the surface of the bones which has the beneficial effect, not the part lodged within the bony tissue. This is why you need to go on taking the tablets.

Effects on the bone

If you are under about 45 when you start taking a bisphosphonate the resorption of bone speeds up initially, but later slows down, and there is an increase in bone formation. After a short time the resorption and formation run in synchrony again, but at a slower rate than before you began the medication. Bone loss continues at a much reduced rate. Your back and your wrists are the bones most affected at this age.

If you are in the older age bracket – 45 to all the way – the rate of resorption slows down from the start, and the bones involved most are the hips, the vertebrae, shoulders, lower leg bones and the pelvis. Bone turnover is generally slowed so that bone formation lags behind resorption, the more so as you get older. Although there is no upper age limit for taking bisphosphonates (unlike HRT) the joint effects of age and the drug may slow turnover so much that it almost comes to a halt. This requires a reduction in the daily dose.

Another danger is that if bone resorption is suppressed too efficiently and for too long by the bisphosphonate it may induce the suppression of bone formation secondarily. In higher doses bisphosphonates prevent the mineralization of bone (the incorporation of calcium which provides its strength). Both these factors may lead to an increased risk of fracture. A lesser worry is the possible long-term effect of having the drug trapped within the bones for years, but to date no one has found any disturbance of the bone metabolism due to this.

Intermittent treatment

Some specialists favour giving bisphosphonates intermittently rather than continuously, with a view to avoiding the stage when bone formation as well as resorption is cut back. In one important study, phosphate was given first to stimulate osteoclast activity, followed by two weeks on etidronate and then 70 days with no treatment, repeating the cycle over several months. This regimen certainly produced short-term improvement in bone mass but the long-term effects are uncertain.

Another method is to give the bisphosphonate by infusion into a vein, two days running, every three months. A trial using alendronate led to a 9 per cent increase in BMD after 12 months. A similar regime with pamidronate, another bisphosphonate being studied, showed increases of 10.5 and 4.5 per cent in different areas of bone after two years. Similar but lesser increases in bone density resulted from taking pamidronate and alendronate tablets by mouth.

One essential when you are on any bisphosphonate is to take sufficient calcium every day. If your diet does not easily provide enough you will need a calcium supplement – tablets or drink – but you must take it at a different time from the bisphosphonate, and not within half an hour. It is ideal to have the latter first thing in the morning and the calcium last thing at night, when it will anyway have the most beneficial effect.

Reminder

When you are starting on either etidronate or alendronate be sure to tell your doctor of any digestive troubles you have had, past or present, including gastritis, duodenal or gastric ulcer, or inflammation of the gullet – oesophagitis. It is also important to mention any kidney problems, and list any medicines you take, including those you buy over the counter. If, after you have started on the bisphosphonate, you find you have heartburn which is getting worse, pain behind the breastbone or discomfort with swallowing, stop the tablets and consult your doctor. Do not take an indigestion medicine.

Drug interactions

There are no harmful interactions with any of the common medicines, but calcium supplements, antacids and various other medicines taken by mouth may interfere with the absorption of the bisphosphonate. Nothing else should be taken within half an hour of the drug.

Side-effects

These are seldom a problem with the two bisphosphonates currently licensed for the treatment of osteoporosis: etidronate and alendronate. Pamidronate has been withdrawn because it produced an unacceptable number of side-effects, that is in one in ten people or more. The small risk of side-effects is minimized if you avoid taking the tablets late in the evening; if you have forgotten to take them in the morning the latest time must be before supper, remembering that you need to have had nothing going into your stomach in the previous hour.

The commonest side-effects are in the digestive system: abdominal discomfort or pain, dyspepsia, constipation or diarrhoea, bloating and wind, and discomfort on swallowing. Others are headache and joint pains.

Even less common are nausea, heartburn, inflammation of the gullet and a rash.

Infusions into a vein can cause local irritation and a transient rise in body temperature.

Precautions

- Do not take the tablet last thing at night.
- Do not chew or suck the tablet – swallow it quickly with the water.
- Do not lie down until you have had something to eat and this should not be sooner than half an hour after taking the tablet. If you are not able to remain vertical for a full half-hour this medication is not for you.

What happens when you stop the treatment?

Does starting on bisphosphonates mean the beginning of a life sentence? Is it disastrous to stop? In two studies, no further bone loss occurred in people, six months and two years respectively after they gave up the medication. This sounds reassuring but is not much use if it does not also mean a reduction in the risk of fractures. Theoretically, an increase of 10 per cent in bone mass should reduce the risk by 50 per cent, but bone mass is not the only relevant factor. BMD is far more important, and only small increases in this, for instance due to HRT, cause a definite decrease in the number of fractures.

An existing fracture is a major risk factor for further fractures, regardless of the bone mass. A study of bisphosphonate treatment over six years in people with previous vertebral crush fractures resulted in their having little or no further loss of height – so no further fractures. This is particularly good news for the vast number of women, mainly, who have begun to develop an ugly stoop.

Currently the pharmaceutical companies are beavering away, trying to come up with the perfect bisphosphonate – one that increases bone strength throughout the skeleton, particularly in long-established osteoporosis, stimulates bone formation as well as reducing resorption, and has negligible side-effects. Already the benefits conferred by these drugs include an increase in BMD in 96 per cent of patients, with a corresponding reduction in risk of fractures. The number of hip fractures, for instance, is down by 63 per cent after 18 months on alendronate tablets.

Winifred

Winifred, 65, was recently retired from the Post Office where she had worked for 35 years. She was looking forward to playing more golf, but meanwhile she had got a new flat, nearer her nephew and his wife. She had probably overdone things humping boxes about during the move – now she had a nasty stabbing pain between her shoulder blades. It was still nagging her a fortnight later, so she went along to the doctor. A plain X-ray showed osteoporosis of the spine, so he checked her history.

The plus points were that Winifred had never smoked, barely touched alcohol and took a healthy amount of exercise on the golf course. She had never married or borne a child and had both a late menarche (first period) and an early menopause, at 41. This made it likely that she was low on oestrogen and apparently an ideal case for HRT. However, her mother had died at the age of 58 from cancer of the womb, which made hormone treatment too risky. Yet she definitely needed effective treatment: a bone densitometry test and a calcium estimation showed that the BMD of her spine was low and her calcium level also below average.

She needed to rev up her calcium intake and the doctor prescribed Adcal, one of the calcium and vitamin D preparations. She took this after lunch and after supper. Calcium alone would not be enough to treat her osteoporosis effectively and calcitonin is awkward to take, so her doctor suggested Fosamax (alendronate). Winifred read the instructions carefully.

She took the round white 10 mg tablet as soon as she woke up, washing it down with a full glass of water from the tap. She got dressed at once, thinking that would usefully fill in the half-hour during which she had to stay upright and must not eat or drink. In fact it did not take that long and she bent about rather freely getting her clothes on, and she was surprised to find that she was getting some burning discomfort in her chest. Her first thought was to take a dose of indigestion medicine – her favourite was Gaviscon – but checking with her doctor he said certainly not, and that medicines containing aluminium were the worst.

He advised her to use a kitchen timer to make sure of staying upright for – he suggested – 40 minutes, and to remember the upright posture while she put her clothes on. Her breakfast, a huge mug of milky coffee and muesli with yoghurt, was full of calcium, but taken late enough not to impair the absorption of the alendronate.

Winifred's low bone mass, 2.4 SD (standard deviations) below the norm, made it a certainty that she would have had further fractures in her vertebrae and perhaps other bones without treatment. After the initial hiccup with the medication, Winifred had no more problems and continued on the daily dose for nine months. Her BMD improved and her bone mass was now only 1.5 SD under par. The pain subsided during the first three or four months, blessedly, but golf, with its spine-twisting movements, is no longer the best type of exercise for her. Walking is always safe, so Winifred is planning a holiday exploring – on foot.

Recent advances in treatment

The last four or five years have been remarkable for the advances in the treatment of osteoporosis. The advent of the bisphosphonates was a major step. Etidronate (Didronel) was the first of them, followed by alendronate (Fosamax Once Weekly), then risedronate (Actonel Once-a-Week). The latter two are both 100 times as potent as Didronel, with a dosage of 35 mg weekly or 10 mg daily for treatment, and 5 mg daily as a preventative. There is nothing to choose between them in efficacy but the side-effects may differ. These are not common or severe but include stomach upsets and pain, a sore tongue and oesophagus or food tube, and headache.

Forsteo (teriparatide)

While the bisphosphonates act by slowing down the rate of removal of older bone, resorption, by cells called osteoclasts, teriparatide has a different action. It increases the rate of bone repair and replacement by stimulating the osteoblasts or bone-building cells. The bone density or strength is increased, lessening the risk of fracture of vertebrae, hip or wrist. Spinal (vertebral) fractures are reduced by 65–69 per cent and others by 35–40 per cent through the use of Forsteo, and the beneficial results continue up to 31 months after stopping treatment. A course of treatment takes 18 months, and this should not be exceeded because of a few cases of sarcoma (a type of cancer) in animals on long-term treatment.

Forsteo is given once daily by a 20 micrograms (mcg) subcutaneous injection (just under the skin) by the patient herself, using a syringe similar to that used in insulin-controlled diabetes. Possible side-effects include nausea, dizziness, leg cramps, anaemia or depression. The improvement in bone density may then be maintained by alternative anti-osteoporosis treatments: SERMs such as raloxifene, or one of the bisphosphonates. Supplements of calcium and vitamin D may be required if the serum levels are low.

Strontium ranelate

Strontium ranelate, provisional trade-name Protelos, was launched in the UK in 2005. It is the first in a new class of drug for osteoporosis which has a double mechanism for strengthening the bones and reducing the risk of fractures. It suppresses the osteoclasts which break down old bone and stimulates the bone-building osteoblasts. So far no studies have been completed comparing Protelos with other drugs in osteoporosis, though it appears that it is equally efficacious in reducing the risk of vertebral fractures but may not work as well for hips and wrists. However, its use is currently recommended for reducing the risk of both spinal and hip fractures.

Side-effects with Protelos are mild, very few, and short-lived. The most common are nausea and diarrhoea, usually in the first few days of treatment. A study in *The New England Journal of Medicine* by Dr Pierre J. Meunier et al. compared the effects of Protelos with those of a placebo, a preparation that is inert medically.

In this study 1,649 postmenopausal women with osteoporosis, who had each suffered at least one vertebral fracture, were randomly divided into two groups: one on placebo, the other on 2 g of Protelos daily. Both were taking supplements of calcium and vitamin D. The trial lasted three years. The results were that the risk of new vertebral fractures was reduced by 49 per cent in the first year of treatment and 41 per cent over the whole three-year period. Bone density, a measure of its strength, was increased at 36 months by 14.4 per cent in the lower spine and 8.3 per cent in the neck of the femoral bone, the hip. There were no serious side-effects in either Protelos or placebo groups. The conclusions from the study are: 'Treatment of postmenopausal osteoporosis with strontium ranelate leads to early and sustained reduction in the risk of vertebral fractures.'

Finally, Southampton and Nottingham Universities have each received funding for research into growing replacement bone in the laboratory. This could kick-start recovery from osteoporosis.

10

Getting over a broken hip and other fractures

Hip fracture

A fractured hip is a major event in anybody's book, but it need not be a disaster.

The cause is osteoporosis and in 90 per cent of cases the trigger is a fall. This is usually nothing dramatic – no further than from a standing position on to level ground. The odd 10 per cent of hip fractures may be due to an unwise twisting movement – you turn round to see where you are going when you are backing the car, or you reach round to pick something up behind you. Sometimes there is no definite precipitant – osteoporosis has made the bone so frail that it just gives way, spontaneously. On the other hand, not all falls in the over-sixties lead to a hip fracture. In fact only two per cent do. The nub is: why does it happen in these cases?

What makes a fall injurious?

- Falling on to your side, on or near your hip joint.
- Walking slowly so that you tend to fall backwards. If you trip when walking briskly your forward momentum makes you tend to fall forwards – you may break your wrist but you save your hip with your outstretched hands.
- The severity of the fall, for example down steps or a slope.
- Age over 75: your reaction time may not be quick enough for you to save yourself.
- Weak triceps and other upper arm muscles so that you may not be strong enough to grab hold of anything effectively.
- Small, thin type of person, so there is not much natural padding over your hip.
- Tall type – you have further to fall.
- Hard, slippery surface to fall on.
- Common home hazards: loose rugs, trailing wires, inadequate (? economical) lighting.
- Previous fracture, anywhere, raises the odds by 20 per cent.
- The size and shape of the bones. This varies from individual to individual, race to race and by sex. Men's bones are generally bigger and more robust.
- A longer than average neck of the femur is a weak point.

- Bone strength, measured by bone mass and bone mineral density: the lower the figures the more vulnerable the bones, due in turn to increasing age, cigarettes, too much alcohol, or poor nutrition or malabsorption with a lack of calcium or vitamin D.

'It happened so quickly!'

Youngsters – say in their sixties and seventies – usually trip or slip over a loose mat or the like. Oldies, from 80 to 90-plus, more often have drop attacks, dizzy turns, faints (syncope), or lose their balance.

Loss of balance

The sense of balance tends to fall off over the years, just as we tend to lose some of our acuity of hearing. The organs of hearing and balance are both in one package, in your ear. Risky times are getting out of bed in the morning and going to the loo.

Drop attacks

These are disconcerting events in which you suddenly find yourself on the ground, but can get up again immediately (unless you have broken your hip), fully conscious. They are due to a transient shortage of blood in the area of the brain stem concerned with posture.

Positive factors

These may surprise you:

- Being slightly overweight, natural padding.
- Osteoarthritis or osteoarthrosis of the hip, because the bone round the joint is thickened.

The fall

You trip, slip or miss your footing, or just fall down, and you have a pain in your hip – sharp or penetrating or a super-ache. Usually you know that you cannot get up and to move your thigh at all is agony. If you do manage to drag yourself up, or someone helps you, you cannot bear the slightest weight on the bad side. Very occasionally the broken parts are wedged together and you can hobble after a fashion and may not realize what has happened.

Obviously you must get to a hospital ASAP. Appropriately you qualify as both an accident and an emergency. There they will examine you including an X-ray and tell you the diagnosis – broken hip.

Types of hip fracture

They are divided into three categories by the position of the break (see diagram on p. 14):

1 *Cervical or intracapsular*: that is, through the neck of the thigh bone (femur) within the capsule, the tough membrane enclosing the joint.
2 *Trochanteric or intertrochanteric, or extracapsular*: between the greater and lesser trochanters, two bumps in the bone where the neck comes off. They are outside the joint capsule.
3 *Subtrochanteric*: below the trochanters, near the top of the shaft of the femur.

Although what you feel when the break happens is much the same whichever the site, there are important differences which will affect the treatment.

The peak age for a hip fracture is 75, but the range runs from around 40 to the nineties and onwards. The under-sixties are likely to have a particular reason for their fractures, and these include:

- removal of the ovaries, usually in with a hysterectomy;
- an early menopause;
- long-term steroid medication;
- anorexia nervosa or other causes of severe malnutrition;
- intolerance of dairy products, with a lack of calcium;
- some forms of cancer.

Some people run short of calcium or perhaps vitamin D without ever realizing that there is any risk to their bones.

Malcolm

Malcolm was 60 when he had the distinction of being one of the few men – compared with women – to fracture his hip. It was not that he suffered a horrific accident. All he had done was to fall off his bike sideways when he had to stop suddenly behind a car. Malcolm had never been keen on sport, except on television, and his job was sedentary, but he had to do a lot of entertaining. This fitted in with his tastes admirably. He was not into what he termed 'nursery food' – milk, ice cream, yogurt, ordinary cheddar and 'green stuff'. He went for a diet based on steak and chips washed down with lager, while his favourite evening tipple was Glenfiddich.

The bike accident left him with a cervical fracture of his left hip. It was repaired by a multiple pinning operation. While he was in hospital he ran into some frightening alcohol withdrawal symptoms. This made it easier for his wife and the doctor to get him to cut back on the booze, which had, after all, been partly responsible for the weakness of his bones. He has also been persuaded to have less red meat, but more fish and cheese – he enjoys a good Stilton. His well-wishers have failed, however, on the exercise front. Malcolm cannot face taking, say, a short daily walk – and he uses his hip as his excuse! The bone has knitted well round the pins and he has very little discomfort.

Exercise would be an insurance against further fractures.

Cervical fractures

These occur most often in the younger group – women in their fifties upwards and men from their sixties. The plus factors for these fractures are that the bone is not usually comminuted – smashed in pieces – and there is seldom any serious bleeding. What there is is contained within the capsule. The broken surfaces of bone may have remained in alignment and in that case are likely to heal well – that was the situation in Malcolm's case. His comparative youth was a plus point, too.

A less favourable scenario is where the broken parts are displaced. There is a substantial risk that the blood vessels to the head of the femur will have been injured. The hip joint is of a ball-and-socket design with the head of the femur as the ball. If there is damage to its vital blood supply, the tissues may not be able to survive, and begin to suffer localized death – 'avascular necrosis'. This means that the first operation, aimed at stabilizing the joint so that healing can take place, has failed. The only option is a second, more radical operation: either hemiarthroplasty (see p. 79) or total hip replacement.

Trochanteric fractures

On the face of it you might think these would fare worse than the cervical type since the victim is usually older and the bone likely to be broken into pieces: a comminuted fracture. In fact these breaks heal better, partly because the bone in this area is of the trabecular type, and more active and amenable. The cervical bone, by contrast, is mainly hard, unchanging cortex – more difficult to smash but less conducive to mending and remodelling.

A disadvantage of the trochanteric type of fracture used to be its propensity to haemorrhage.

Subtrochanteric fractures

These are the least common. They are often comminuted and even more difficult to stabilize than the trochanteric sort. They are likely to require complex arrangements of plates and screws, with skilled insertion. This procedure is liable to be complicated by bleeding at the time.

Treatment of hip fracture

It is urgent – and surgical – but whichever operation your orthopaedic surgeon decides on, the preliminaries are the same. Some time after you are settled in bed, your anaesthetist will check you over with particular attention to your chest, heart and blood pressure. Nowadays, keyhole surgery means very little injury.

The operations

Hemiarthroplasty

This is the standard operation for an intracapsular fracture, especially if there is displacement or any damage to the blood supply to the joint. It is a must if there is a threat of avascular necrosis, a crumbling of the bone due to lack of blood. It consists of fitting a *prosthesis*, an artificial replacement for a part, for instance like false teeth. In this case the prosthesis replaces the head of the femur. There are two provisos: the hip must not have been damaged by arthritis, nor must the joint socket show signs of wear and tear. In these situations the bigger operation of total hip replacement – socket and all – is the best recourse.

Both these operations have the advantage of allowing almost immediate mobility with full weight-bearing on the affected side. On the other hand, they are major procedures and a replacement joint is never quite as flexible and adaptable as a completely healed natural hip joint. Nor do the prostheses last indefinitely and they may need replacing when you are older and less fit. In fragile bone the prosthesis may be fixed in place with a special cement. More recently a porous metal is used which allows the bone to grow into it. This method is indicated if you are younger and active, and your bones are still fairly strong.

Internal fixation

This is a lesser operation than fitting a half (hemi-) or total hip prosthesis and is usually employed in trochanteric fractures to fix the pieces of bone in position. There are three types of internal fixation:

1 *Multiple pins* or screws: usually three are required, going into the head of the femur. They are mainly used for cervical fractures.
2 *Dynamic hip screws* or 'sliding hip nails': one or more large nails or screws fixing a steel plate across the fracture. They are used for extracapsular, trochanteric breaks.
3 *Intramedullary device*: a rod is inserted in the middle of the femur, from the shaft into the head, and fixed with screws. This operation is used for subtrochanteric fractures in particular. Operations depending on pinning

the broken parts take longer to heal than replacement surgery because the damaged tissues are not removed. These may be extensive.

The younger and livelier you are, the more likely your surgeon is to suggest a pinning operation, while if you are definitely elderly, total hip replacement straight off may be the best option. As a senior you are likely to have some arthritis and may well require this operation in due course anyway. Recovery from hemiarthroplasty or total hip replacement provides the quickest route back to walking, an important consideration in older people, who do not cope well with being off their feet for a day longer than necessary.

Complications of hip surgery

Complications necessitating a second operation occur in about a third of internal fixation operations. Hemiarthroplasty and total hip replacement lead to far fewer problems and less pain during the recovery period. Non-union, a failure of the broken bone to join up within a reasonable period, is the likeliest snag, with avascular necrosis one step worse. Joint infection after the fitting of a prosthesis may relate back to some pre-existing condition. Chest and urinary infections and clotting in a leg vein (deep vein thrombosis, DVT) may crop up after any operation involving time in bed.

Maggie

Maggie was 48, and it was five years since her hysterectomy and oophorectomy (ovary removal) for cancer of the cervix. She was now well, and beginning to be less anxious about the possibility of a relapse – until she broke her left hip, getting off a bus. At first she and her doctor were afraid this was due to a secondary cancer, but the X-ray was reassuring. Maggie did not have arthritis and normally enjoyed an active life, so it was decided to do an internal fixation with multiple pins. A biopsy, among other tests, confirmed that she did not have bone cancer, but showed established osteoporosis. This was not surprising, with her early surgical menopause and no HRT cover, because of the cancer.

The fracture, a trochanteric type, needed urgent surgical treatment. With an extracapsular fracture and her young age, internal fixation was the operation of choice and the type chosen was multiple pinning. Unfortunately after a few weeks Maggie's hip became increasingly painful, until she was unable to put her foot to the ground on that side. X-rays showed that the bone had failed to unite across the break and the screws were working loose. A hemiarthroplasty was then carried out and Maggie's progress has since been positive and untroubled.

After your operation

The overriding objective is mobilization, but in the early days your main concern will be the damping down of the pain. At first you will have powerful painkillers such as morphine or pethidine by injection. One neat little apparatus allows you to inject yourself, as and when you feel the need, through a tube fixed into a wrist vein. It is arranged so that you cannot overdose yourself.

The need for strong analgesia only lasts a few days, and then you can cope with milder drugs, like paracetamol. You may have a daily suppository of one of the anti-inflammatories (NSAIDs) to tide you over the transition, and perhaps the luxury of an icepack on the joint area. You will feel better in yourself when you are off the morphine. It is difficult to get your head together while you are taking it, and most people get waves of nausea and may occasionally vomit. Now, while you are in hospital, and for some weeks afterwards, you will need to get used to sleeping on your back and remembering not to cross your legs, not even at the ankle. You must not put the slightest twisting strain on the joint.

While you are concerned with these day-to-day details your hip is already beginning to mend. Your job is to help it in every way.

Exercise is the key

From the moment you come round from the anaesthetic you can start:

- breathing exercises, not forgetting to use your diaphragm;
- shrugging your shoulders;
- tensing your leg and thigh muscles as though you were trying to make the limb perfectly straight;
- screwing up and stretching out your toes; do the same with your hands;
- rolling your ankles round and pointing your toes down and then up;
- lifting your arms forwards and sideways;
- pressing your bottom muscles together;
- turning your head from side to side.

You can do all of these lying flat. Within 24 hours the physiotherapist, looking fit and strong, will bear down on you. She or he will teach and encourage you all through your hospital stay with a progressive series of exercises. The emphasis is on encouragement, because she will constantly be asking you to do what seems impossible, beginning by standing out of bed the day after your operation, when you have had a total replacement or hemiarthroplasty. Somehow you will do what she asks. Remember what we do to little children – getting them to believe that they can stand on their own two feet, then totter a few steps with help, although their legs are weak and wobbly and out of control. It is much the same after a hip operation.

The exercises the physio will show you, for example lifting your leg off the bed, and moving your hip in different ways, are pure gold. They will stand you in good stead literally for years to come. You will be helped to walk at first with a Zimmer frame, then two elbow sticks, then two without elbow pieces – then one. The latter stages will be after you have left hospital and finally you may be able to manage with no stick. However, before you go home you will have a crash course in negotiating stairs. It may not be the quickest or most elegant way of going up or down, but it gets you there safely.

One of the most enjoyable moments of your hospital stay is when you give up wearing the hideous, white, uncomfortably compressive anti-thrombosis stockings. They feel worse in summer, but they are important. A clot forming in a vein (DVT) is a painful and potentially dangerous complication of surgery. You may be given heparin by injection to reduce the risk further.

Going home

You are likely to stay in hospital between 3 and 4 days. When you leave you will need two sticks, adjusted for your height, and a type of rigid plastic ring to raise the level of your loo seat. Bending at the hip remains difficult, and it hurts, for weeks to come. This is the limiting factor which makes it difficult for you to get in or out of a car, sit in a low chair or get up from it, put your shoes and socks on, or pick something up off the floor.

I say *socks* because putting on tights or stockings seems to require the contortions of an acrobat. You will not be up to that for some weeks yet, and a longish skirt with an elasticated waist is easier to get into than jeans. Fortunately there are tools that help: an ingenious plastic affair for socks, a long shoehorn – preferably wear shoes fastening with Velcro – and a 'helping hand' which enables you to grab everything that ends up on the floor. This last is extremely useful, even in your 'after-life', for getting hold of articles which are awkward to reach.

Shopping

Now you are back home you must be like a general, planning your strategy. Fine if you have a willing, live-in relative such as a husband, but today so many of us live on our own. Right away you have to work out how you are going to get your shopping, since you do not want to add starvation to your problems. Ordering on the Internet may not be practicable for a household of one, and personally I divided my needs among my neighbours so that none had to fetch more than one or two items. I got on to the happiest terms with them all, including those I hardly knew before. As I lived upstairs and it took me forever to go up or down, we evolved a super system of my lowering a basket from my window when anyone rang my bell to announce the arrival of supplies.

Cooking

This involves standing, which is bad for your hip and causes a painful dragging feeling. Plan to have hot drinks, since lifting a kettle is no great problem, but otherwise nothing that requires preparation. Heating in a microwave is the most you should attempt for many weeks to come.

Nourishment

The insult to your body of the fracture and the surgery will have left it depleted of protein, and with a need for building up in general. Cheese, tofu and sardines provide both protein and calcium; fruit and salads give you vitamin C, needed for the healing process; okra, a big orange and curly kale contain calcium as well as vitamin C. See p. 105 for full details on diet.

Driving

Once you have mastered sliding in behind the steering wheel you are set to go if you have an automatic. You only need one good leg and it does not matter which. You may be able to drive within six weeks, but a little longer if you have a manual gear change. This may be the time to consider getting a blue disabled badge. It allows you to park in special, convenient slots in most car parks and if necessary to stop on a yellow line. This may be essential for shopping or keeping in touch with other people. Your GP will know the ropes locally and may have to provide a letter.

Exercise

Establish the habit of a morning and/or evening stint of the exercises your physio has suggested. This way you will reduce morning stiffness, pain and general weakness – the effort truly pays off. Outdoor exercise, basically walking, is a tonic which includes self-made vitamin D, and, to start with, a sense of adventure. The trick is to go a little further every day – for starters I could only manage to get to the first lamp-post down my road. See p. 103 for the general purpose exercise regime.

All this may sound impossibly ambitious. It is well within your reach if you were fighting fit before the accident, but many of us need a spell in a rehabilitation ward or other facility. This may be the moment to rearrange your living accommodation and perhaps move into sheltered housing, a home for the elderly or a nursing home. A third of us find that we are more dependent after a hip fracture, but in any event, you can expect your health and strength to improve progressively so long as you do four things:

1 Take what exercise you are able to manage, hopefully to include walking, but bed exercise if that is all that is within your range at present.

2 Have nourishing meals; eating even when you are not hungry will help a poor appetite to grow.

3 Take calcium and vitamin D supplements and other medicines with your doctor's approval.

4 See your friends as much as they can happily manage, and build in at least one 'treat' every week, so that you always have something to look forward to. Depression is the bugbear of the pain and frustration of having broken your hip – zap it in advance. You may like to join an osteoporosis group, often combined with arthritis, as a social outing where you can compare notes and perhaps pick up useful tips from fellow sufferers.

You must avoid the following:

- sitting with your hips lower than your knees;
- squatting;
- bending your hip joint more than 90 degrees;
- jarring your joints by running, however slowly, or jumping down a step, however low;
- swimming breast stroke (see p. 103).

Michael

Ever since his retirement four years before, Michael had taken a daily 'constitutional' – a walk for health and pleasure. One of his favourite routes was through an oak wood with many fine trees. He blamed his new glasses, but it was already getting dusk when he caught his foot in a spreading root. He fell heavily and realized at once that he had broken his hip. All he could do was to remain on the ground until someone came that way. He had not carried his mobile when he was only going for an evening stroll.

Fortunately Michael did not have very long to wait before a young couple came through the trees, and the complicated rescue began. X-rays revealed a cervical fracture with the broken surfaces out of line – and osteoporosis. Pinning was impracticable, so that left hemiarthroplasty or total hip replacement as the choices. Michael's joints were already showing signs of wear-and-tear osteoarthritis, so the better option was a full hip replacement. He had no chronic illness, but in the past he had sustained two fractures from playing rugby: these would have depleted his bone mass.

True to his nature, Michael was determined to get fit as soon as possible. He was out of bed the day after his operation and walking with a Zimmer two days later. He worked hard at the exercises and made a sparkling recovery, walking half a mile every day (no sticks) and driving his car again within a month of getting home. Not everyone can expect to manage as well as Michael: his general condition before the operation was excellent for a man of 69.

He has now started a new regimen with daily exercise, calcium and vitamin supplements, and shoes with non-slip soles instead of the smooth leather he had always preferred. It is useless, however, to tell his grandchildren not to make the sitting room floor into an obstacle course of abandoned toys.

Your home, too, may contain hazards for your hips and other joints. Falls are a big danger, so you need to know the best ways of avoiding them (see Chapter 11).

Other fractures from osteoporosis

Colles' fracture of the wrist

One in five women of 70 in the UK and the US have already had a broken wrist. The number who suffer from a Colles' fracture (see p. 16) escalates from the start of the menopause, reaching a peak between 60 and 70. It levels off then, but is more serious when it affects an older person. Most victims who are over 85 will need hospitalization. Although it is not life-threatening, a fractured wrist is very painful. Setting the fracture is tricky and may have to be repeated more than once, and it requires four to six weeks in plaster to heal.

A troublesome long-term effect, lasting a year or more, is *algodystrophy*. This arises in about a third of cases, and causes the wrist to remain painful, swollen and tender to pressure. Carpal tunnel syndrome or a frozen shoulder may develop secondarily. Pain relief and physiotherapy are your main concern and often a complementary treatment will help, for example aromatherapy.

Shoulder fracture

A fall jarring your whole arm or an impact on your shoulder may cause a break where the head of the humerus, the long bone in your upper arm, joins the shaft. This is rather similar to a trochanteric hip fracture.

If you are lucky the bone will heal in about four weeks if the joint is immobilized. It is only after this that the real hard work begins. It can take months of physiotherapy and exercise to restore full movement. Doing your hair is the most difficult action. As with a hip fracture, the blood supply to the head of the bone may be damaged – with the same outcome: avascular necrosis. The answer is similar, too – a hemiarthrosis, replacing the head of the humerus in this case. Pinning is usually unsuccessful, but the replacement operation makes the joint mobile almost immediately. Pain is not usually too bad.

Shin-bone fracture

The tibia, or shin-bone, is topped by a flattish surface which forms part of the knee joint.

Stella

When she was 50 Stella broke the top of her tibia in the classic way by stepping off the kerb with a bump. The sudden jarring pressure with her whole weight behind it drove some of the upper surface of the bone into the spongy, cancellous part underneath. The injured bone healed but Stella's knee was painful and unstable. Fortunately knee replacement operations are now standard in the bigger orthopaedic centres. Stella's new knee is a success, and she is working to check any worsening of her osteoporosis.

Ankle fracture

We get broken ankles at all ages, including middle age and older, with osteoporosis. Usually the break heals satisfactorily in a walking plaster, all the better because of the pressure on it. Healing is delayed if you rest up. If there is displacement of the fracture, the loose piece is fixed in position with screws. Recovery is straightforward.

Metatarsal fracture

You can easily break one of these foot bones by stepping into a hole unawares or twisting your foot. The fracture heals well, needing only strapping to ease the pain and provide support.

Backbone fractures

Neck or cervical vertebrae

A break in one of these bones is rarely due to osteoporosis, but the cause needs urgent investigation.

Chest or thoracic vertebrae

These are the bones most subject to compression fractures in osteoporosis, leading to the exaggerated stoop, kyphosis, unkindly called dowager's hump. It may develop or worsen without your feeling anything, but on the other hand you may get acute back pain without there being any definite break to be seen on the X-ray.

Lower back or lumbar vertebrae

These, too, are frequently affected by osteoporosis, usually causing chronic backache. You cannot relieve thoracic or lumbar back pain by splinting, but bed rest, however much it beckons, is not the answer. It involves the risk of venous thrombosis (clot in a vein) and is liable to make the osteoporosis worse. The best ploy is to keep moving as much as you can, pottering about, and to take painkillers when you need them. The attack always subsides to a large extent in the end.

Loss of height and forward curvature of the spine progresses very slowly, then stops when the lowest ribs touch the hip bones. This can be uncomfortable, but becomes less so, with analgesics meanwhile.

See also Chapter 2 for more on backbone fractures.

When you have had the experience of one broken bone, and knowing how easily it can happen, especially for a second time, of course you are afraid of having a fall. The answer is not to try to stay safe by skulking away at home, but to take positive action. Find out all about falls, how they happen and the practical steps you can take to avoid them. It is all in Chapter 11.

11
Falls

Ninety-five per cent of broken bones, at any age, result from a fall, and breaks involve pain, disability and disruption to your life. A Colles' fracture means you cannot drive, do most types of job, clean the house or play the piano, while a hip fracture means a big operation and knocks you off your feet for weeks – at best. It also involves serious risks.

No one plans on having a fall, but it makes good sense to do all you can to avoid such an event – even if you are still in your forties and by no stretch of the imagination doddery. Take it seriously for sure if you are 20 years older, know that you have some of the risk factors or have had an actual diagnosis of osteoporosis. Most important of all, take avoiding action if you have already broken a bone – that increases the risk of a new fracture by 20 per cent.

Are you at risk?

- Are you a woman?
- Are you slim, with no spare flesh as padding?
- Are you taller than average, with farther to fall?
- Are you past the menopause?
- Are you sometimes unsteady on your feet?
- Have you any joint or foot problem which interferes with your gait?
- Do you suffer from either form of arthritis – rheumatoid or osteoarthritis?
- Do you take sleeping tablets?
- Do you have to get up in the night to pass water?
- Have you given up taking much exercise?

All the 'yes's' are negative points – indications that you personally are at some risk of having a fall. The passing years, in either sex, increase this risk.

Women

The risks of at least one fall this year are:

- one in five if you are between 60 and 65;
- one in three if you are between 80 and 85;
- one in two if you are 85 and over.

Men

You are protected by having a larger, heavier frame for starters, and for your sex only, increasing age brings an increase in the width of the individual bones. This applies to all of them, including the hip bones and the vertebrae: the cross-section of the latter can increase by 25 to 30 per cent.

You begin to catch up with the women for vulnerability at 80-plus. The risk of at least one fall in the year is one in three when you reach 85.

Triggers to a fall

- 50 per cent are due to a trip or slip, especially among the under-sixties.
- 20 per cent are due to a faint (syncope), drop attack or other interruption of brain function.
- 20 to 30 per cent are caused by losing your balance.

Naturally, the oldest people are at most risk. If you are among them:

- Drop attacks are common: these consist in a sudden, brief failure of the blood supply to part of the brain, so that you fall to the ground without warning (and cannot save yourself) but recover immediately.
- The postural reflexes slow down so that you do not fling your arms out in time, or swing your body round soon enough to prevent or break your fall.
- The balance organ in your ear is not so efficient these days.
- Your muscles are not so strong now that you are living a gentler life.
- Your blood pressure takes a little longer to respond and send enough blood to your brain when you stand up, so you may feel faint or dizzy when you get up from bed or a chair.
- Some older people do not bother to eat enough and this can leave their brains depleted of sugar.

On a plus point, if you feel swimmy getting up from a chair, you are not likely to hurt yourself even if you fall – it is not far. Similarly, you can feel faint on the loo when you pass water but do not usually come to harm. The more dangerous situations are when you are standing still or walking very slowly, changing direction, reaching for something, or stepping slowly down one step.

Sylvia

Sylvia was 75. Whether she had an evening drink or nothing after 6 p.m., she usually woke once or twice in the night to go to the loo. Occasionally she took a temazepam tablet to help her sleep and it was on one of these occasions that she woke at 2 a.m. and felt slightly dizzy and disorientated on the trip to the bathroom. She was in a hurry to get there in time but her circulation had not had sufficient time to adjust to her being upright after three-and-a-half hours horizontal. She had begun to move forwards slowly when she fell in a heap. This time she was only shaken up and slightly bruised.

Now Sylvia waits for a few minutes sitting on the edge of the bed before she stands up. Since she is anxious in case her bladder will not be able to wait she has taken to wearing an incontinence pad at night, for safety's sake.

Checklist of risk factors

Medicines that can make you faint or dizzy

- Sleeping tablets, such as temazepam.
- All types of tranquillizers, from diazepam to chlorpromazine.
- Antidepressants, such as Surmontil or Seroxat.
- Blood pressure medicines, such as Hypovase (prazocin).
- Water tablets of the 'loop' type, like Burinex, which act super-fast. (These last two can lower your blood pressure too much.)
- Tablets for diabetes such as Glibenese (glipizide) which can leave your brain depleted of sugar.
- Digoxin, which slows the heart, and other heart medicines.

Physical problems

- Arthritis or rheumatism.
- Parkinson's disease.
- Foot disorders.
- TIA – transient ischaemic attacks – brief periods of shortage of blood to the brain with furred-up arteries.
- Heart disease.
- Poor vision from cataracts and other causes.
- Depression, slowing you down physically as well as mentally.

Environment – outdoors

- Ice, snow, wet pavements.
- Uneven ground.
- Slippery surfaces.
- Steep slopes.
- Unfamiliar places.
- Getting on and off buses, trains.
- Steps, stairs and escalators.
- Crowds.

Hazards at home

- Loose rugs and carpets, especially stair carpet.
- Wet or highly polished floors.
- Trailing wires.
- Low tables, stools and chairs.
- Clutter so there is no room to move.
- Soft, low chairs without arms.
- Poor lighting, especially on landings.
- Bed too high or too low.

Personal

- Shoes too big, especially slip-ons, insecure fastening, high heels, slippery soles.
- Long skirt you may trip over, going upstairs.
- Trouser legs too long.
- Wearing the wrong glasses.
- Walking stick the wrong height.

Prevention – positive action

- Clear the risk factors above that apply to your home.
- Discuss with your doctor, if you are taking several medicines, to find out if they are all necessary, or if the dosage could be reduced.
- Eat enough good food to prevent any tendency to lose weight, with special care for calcium and vitamins.
- Build up your muscle strength with exercise (see pp. 102–3): those from a physiotherapist, walking and swimming.
- Practise walking briskly – good for your bones and less harmful if you fall.
- If you have a specific walking problem, for example from Parkinsonism, take some exercises to improve your gait.
- Balance exercises from a physiotherapist, if balance is your problem.
- Particularly if your balance is insecure and your confidence is shaky, try the polyurethane hip protectors. They may not be glamorous, but in a recent American trial the number of hip fractures was whittled down by between one half and two-thirds for those wearing these pads. They reduce the impact on the hip by 20 per cent.
- Lastly, build some positive treats into your programme – but not the same as Ben's.

Ben

When Ben was 68 he spent a lot of time in his garden, which gave him a thirst. The pipe had a similar effect. In the evenings he went to the Red Lion to have a drink with his mates, his pipe as ever in his mouth. What he did not realize was that when you get older you cannot metabolize alcohol as efficiently as when you were in your forties. Nor did it occur to him that his bones had been harmed by a lifetime of beer and tobacco. When he was coming home on a frosty evening he slipped and fell against his own gatepost, breaking his right shoulder. It healed fairly well over the next five or six weeks, but his particular grouse was that he could not lift a tankard without pain for months afterwards. Ben's fall was due to one of the top causes – for men!

12

Moods and emotions

Of course your bones are important; they are the framework of your body. But the real you matters a million times more – the way you think, what you feel, your loves and fears, and how you react to what life brings – including osteoporosis.

Stress and depression in themselves impinge on the well-being of your bones and worsen the risks of osteoporosis.

Stress is universal. You cannot escape it and at different times in your life it can centre on money, relationships, work – or health. Emotional stress leads to an outflow of cortisone, your home-made steroid, as damaging to your bones as steroid medication. It causes loss of bone mass, lowers BMD and interferes with the absorption of calcium. Anti-stress manoeuvres are nature's tranquillizers – sharing with a partner, friends and colleagues; the countryside, music, novels, television – and the uncritical companionship of your dog or cat. Physical exercise is a great DIY reducer of stress, and sleep restores you better when you are muscle-tired not worry-weary.

Depression is the bane of all chronic disorders including osteoporosis and, like stress, is itself harmful. Loss of motivation means you do not bother with sensible anti-osteoporosis precautions. Food has lost its savour, which undermines your care for your diet. Interrupted sleep diminishes the time available for tissue repair – essential for your bones if you are over 30. Finally, depression slows you down physically as well as mentally and immobility is death to your bones and muscles. Dealing with depression, as with stress, is important whenever it arises, but since it is a common and understandable reaction to established osteoporosis, it is considered in detail later (see p. 95).

Anxiety

This is a natural response in the early days when the diagnosis of osteoporosis is first mooted, either because of suspicious appearances in an X-ray, an unexpected fracture or a sharp attack of backache. You may be worried to find you have got shorter. Anxiety is next cousin to stress: you cannot relax, get off to sleep or concentrate. It may kill your appetite or by contrast you cannot stop eating, and you are irritable with your nearest and dearest or your workmates. You find yourself brooding about the possible effects of the disease.

Tranquillizing medicines or a few stiff drinks may make you feel better for the time, but they are bad news in the long run. They inevitably lead to depression. Anxiety calls for off-loading, preferably on to a professional, with physical exercise and full-cream milky drinks as your sedatives. When you have taken the edge off your anxiety, find out the facts about osteoporosis – as you are doing now, then have a discussion with your doctor or the practice nurse.

Possible consequences of osteoporosis

Physical	Psychological
Pain, in the back or from a fracture	Stress from coping with difficulties
Reduced activity, enforced	Poor sleep from worry, discomfort
Stooping back, loss of height	Depression, low self-image
Muscle weakness	Feeling worthless, even a nuisance
Easily tired, less energy	Fear for the future
Loss of independence	Feeling angry, helpless

Coping

When your osteoporosis amounts to nothing worse than a little backache and some stiffness, it is a doddle – you are well able to manage. It is a different matter if you get nagging back pain when you stand or sit for too long – say a couple of hours, or when you need to lean forward, for instance at a desk. It becomes increasingly difficult to cope with all your usual activities: driving, carrying shopping, housework, keyboard work or social outings. What makes it worse is that everyone else – family, friends, colleagues – expects you to be the same as you always were. They do not realize that they need to adjust their expectations, just as much as you.

Miriam

Miriam had been a top-rate grandmother when she was in her fifties, her daughter's mainstay in bringing up the first two children. Now Miriam was 64 and she had developed osteoporosis, with crush fractures in her spine which often gave her back pain. She found it hard to explain to her daughter that she simply could not lift Rory, her third grandchild, a fine 30-pound toddler, or even stoop to pick up his toys. She did not have the strength, and it hurt her back. Miriam felt humiliated.

In fact it was not all bad. Miriam's daughter said how nice it was for her and the children to have a granny who behaved like a granny, anchored in one place, and there to read stories and dispense comfort when needed. Her role no longer clashed with the mother's.

Depression

All of us who are in the older generation absolutely hate asking for help from our children – when we have always been the strong, competent ones! A feeling of worthlessness is the fast track to clinical depression. Other symptoms are loss of concentration, a loss of interest in subjects that used to seem important, self-confidence ebbing away, and a tendency to withdrawal, which sets off a vicious circle. A depressed face looks very like a bad-tempered one, and it does not help that you stop caring about your appearance. Nothing pleases you, and everything you say is negative.

Other people misunderstand and may begin to resent your apparent lack of concern. You can come over as uncaring, grumpy and ungrateful. If your osteoporosis gets worse, so does the depression – they are linked. You need help, urgently. One of the best antidepressants for some women after the menopause is HRT (but it is best used only temporarily), for others the standard, modern antidepressants, the SSRIs (selective serotonin re-uptake inhibitors) are better. However, the talking treatments – psychotherapy or simple counselling – are safest and often the most effective. See below.

Beryl

Beryl was 80. She had been a dancer in her youth, admired for her looks and figure. Now she was 5 inches shorter, with a hunched back and, what distressed her most, a stomach that bulged. Cutting down on meals made no difference to that. Beryl said she hated what she had become: old and ugly, and she knew that she was often crotchety. The long days stretched uselessly ahead and although she longed for sleep she would wake in the small hours, fully alert, but long before it was time to get up. Her body was awkward, but not really painful, and her depressed mood was a reaction to her situation rather than a mental illness.

Her daughter Olive could not bear to see Beryl so different from the confident, vibrant woman she used to be and towed her off to the doctor who was busy but efficient. She prescribed alendronate and extra calcium and booked a protesting Beryl in for a course of cognitive therapy with a clinical psychologist. This method of treatment makes antidepressants unnecessary in many cases. Beryl was argued and encouraged out of her habit of automatically seeing the black side and expecting failure at every turn.

The first task was to tot up Beryl's assets, the second to find ways of making use of them, and the third was to add some new elements. All this was a year ago. Now Beryl is working on her memoirs and has joined a local writers' circle where they all help each other. She is valued for her first-hand knowledge of the 1950s and 1960s, and earlier. With a new interest and new contacts Beryl's personality and confidence again began to develop. Her early professional discipline enabled her to get into the way of regular exercise – at home, walking and with a splash in the local swimming pool. Another plus is the understanding and the jokes, which other people cannot appreciate, in the Osteoporosis Group – transport provided.

The final positive change is her constant companion, Hudson, a big black fellow from Cat Rescue. Olive is no longer harassed by the thought of her mother being lonely and miserable.

Adjustment disorder

Everyone with osteoporosis responds in her own way. It may be troublesome enough to impinge on your lifestyle, like other long-term illnesses. The trick is to cultivate a positive attitude towards the inevitable changes, but this is easier said than done. As we get older, say any time after 45, we tend to be less adventurous and prefer what is familiar, but the major hormonal upheaval of the menopause at about 50 ushers in a crowd of other life changes. Your children grow up and your role in relation to them enters a new phase with you no longer in charge. Your own parents are getting older and may, in their turn, need your help and advice. Your partner's health may take a knock, especially if he is some years older than you. Retirement looms.

This stage in your life is like a cross-country race with a series of obstacles to overcome. There is a series of rewards, too, if you look for them. The urgent necessity is past of building up your career or just keeping your job, but now you must adjust your priorities. Plan ahead so that you do not miss out on contacts with old friends or making new ones, seeing your children and grandchildren, of course, and having pleasant interludes even with passing acquaintances.

Assess your physical capacities – what are you able to do? If you can walk 100 yards, aim for 200. If you are near a pool, swim or do any kind of exercise in the water to stimulate your body and boost your muscles. Join any group or club: political, musical or social – the subject does not matter, the people do. See what is on offer at your public library. Finally, make use of the free, constantly available entertainment from TV, radio and the Net. Check through the programme listings so that you can follow up an interest, and be sure to have a coffee at the ready so that you can watch or listen in luxury.

Edna

Edna was not quite 60 when osteoporosis forced her to retire a year or two earlier than she had intended. She had been a hairdresser and could no longer manage being on her feet for so long and bending over the customers' heads. She used not to mind living alone, but now she felt isolated, missing the company and the chatting. To help herself adjust, she joined an over-fifties social club and became an active member of the local Labour Party. The telephone was her lifeline when the weather was bad.

Joan

Joan went through a bad patch just after she broke her hip. She was only 56 and the operation went well, but the timing was dire. Her younger daughter, after a disastrous earlier affair, had found the man of her dreams: at any rate a very nice fellow. Joan was eager to have an active role in the wedding preparations and hobbled round with a stick getting in everyone's way. Trying to do too much too soon, she slipped on the parquet floor and she was afraid she had dislocated her new joint. It was swollen and painful, but the X-ray showed everything still in position. Nevertheless she had got to go carefully.

It was a turning point. Joan did the 'secretarial' work for the wedding, telephoning caterers and answering letters, while the younger generation got on with the energetic tasks. It was a success, so Joan worked out a new life plan for herself with the emphasis on non-physical activities. One small delight was finding she had the knack of writing verses for greetings cards – a minor money-spinner. It helped her through the time while her bruised and battered hip was mending. Afterwards she kept it up for pleasure, and made arrangements to go back to her job in accounts at Trumbles on a part-time basis.

Joan is not mourning for her losses, but meets every change as a challenge – and she is winning.

13

Prevention 1: Lifestyle and exercise

Prevention comes in two packages: the first is the avoidance of osteoporosis altogether – for this you have to start young – and the second is the prevention of its getting worse after it has already begun to develop: this is far the commoner situation.

For your daughter and less importantly – because he is less vulnerable – your son, and for yourself if you are under 25, the top priority is to build a substantial bone mass. By the age of 30 this will be at its maximum, with a trend for very gradual loss of bone from then on. Your peak bone mass is your deposit account, to draw on in need, for instance during pregnancy or after a fracture, rather than for day-to-day fluctuations. The build-up depends on a healthy diet, with plenty of calcium, and a bone-healthy lifestyle.

Diet is vitally important and warrants a chapter to itself (see Chapter 14), while healthy living habits are something you hope to inculcate into your youngster and also to follow yourself – lifelong. Adequate sleep is a must for doing repairs from the wear and tear of your daily activities, but excessive sleeping time – more than eight hours – is counterproductive. So is too much physical rest. Today's youngsters are in particular danger – the attractions of computer games, television and the Net are a threat to their bones.

Lack of movement and exercise has a weakening effect on the trabecular bone in particular, actually altering its internal structure. The two most vulnerable areas are the vertebrae and the neck of the thigh bone. In both of these a small area of trabecular bone carries almost the whole weight of the body.

Of course a good lifestyle includes food for the mind as well as the body: ongoing learning and the inspiration and delight of music, art and literature, plus unashamed entertainment – but these must not crowd out exercise.

What is so special about exercise?

Bone is a living tissue, metabolically active – that is, constantly changing and renewing itself, and exercise is essential for it to do this. Weight-bearing exercise is the only type that stimulates the bone formation part of the endless cycle of removing old tissue, renewing and remodelling it. One of the major problems of space travel is that the astronauts in their weightless environment lose bone at a disastrous rate, and without gravity to work against it is difficult to devise exercises for them that put the necessary pressure on their bones.

No amount of calcium, vitamin D or HRT makes up for lack of weight-bearing exercise. Footballers are more susceptible to stress fractures at the beginning of the season than after a few weeks' training. Similarly with new recruits in the Army – the drill improves their bone strength as well as their muscles. People who live up mountains develop stronger bones than those living on the flat – again, a matter of exercise. Among tennis champions the bone mineral density (BMD) in their dominant arm, the one that hits the aces, is higher than in the other one, while athletes in general have a bone mass 20 to 30 per cent greater than that of sedentary workers.

Exercise may be drastically limited during an illness, with arthritis, or in the case of hemiplegia (partial paralysis) after a stroke, but it is all the more urgent to do whatever you can. In one study, otherwise healthy men who had to rest up while recovering from slipped discs lost BMD in their back bones at the rate of 1 per cent per week, and it took them four months of remobilization to make it up. Disuse leads to resorption, equals loss of bone substance.

It is the repeated stresses and strains on the bones from ordinary living that keeps them up to strength. Four hours on her feet during the day is the minimum necessary to keep a woman's bones healthy, and this definitely cuts the risk of a hip fracture.

Juniors

Your bones go on growing into your late twenties and growing bones are especially responsive to exercise, or the lack of it. Youngsters can benefit their bones with a wide variety of weight-bearing activities: walking, running and dancing; jumping, jogging and skipping; ball games from tennis to hockey to football; athletics and rock-climbing; step aerobics or simply going up and down stairs. It is not all roses, however. Exercise is a two-edged sword.

Too much exercise, for instance for athletic training and in obsessively exercising anorexic girls, suppresses the production of the sex hormones which are needed for strong bones. Girls who have an early menarche (start of periods) have a particularly high bone density with a resistance to fractures, while the opposite is the case with delayed puberty. Athletes and others who go into training before menarche, or the equivalent outflow of testosterone in boys, put their sexual development back by about two years. They never reach their full potential in height, nor achieve as big a bone mass as they would have done. Amenorrhoea – an absence of monthly periods – whenever it occurs, always involves undue bone loss with a high risk of osteoporosis at the time or years later.

Midge

Midge at 11 was the pride of her school, and she was put in for serious athletic training. She was glad not to have the bother of periods when her friends did and they still had not come when she was 16 and in the junior Olympics team. Her particular forte was the high jump and it was in a practice session that she miscalculated and fell awkwardly. She only broke her ankle, but it prevented her from taking part in any athletics for the rest of the season. The X-rays showed her bones looking lacy and transparent from osteoporosis – at 17, although she had been having a generous diet with plenty of calcium.

This was frightening, so her parents, after much heart-searching, pulled her out of competitive athletics. Hormonal treatment gave her periods a jump-start when she was 18, and with graded exercise and an individually planned diet she is making up the lost ground. Her youth is on her side. Of course Midge was upset at losing her status as a sportswoman, but she found herself able to enjoy normal teenage fun when she no longer had to devote so much of her time to training.

Adults

Men are not immune, but it is women who account for 90 per cent of osteoporosis victims and for whom a sensible lifestyle is essential if they are to avoid a load of trouble later. There are traps to avoid, which also apply to men:

Smoking

We all know this is bad for our throat, sinuses and lungs. It is also harmful to our bones, in a round-about way. The menopause starts sooner in smokers, because less oestrogen is produced and it is metabolized more quickly. Fat may be reduced, too – and the fat mass is protective to the bones.

Alcohol

In weekly amounts higher than the recommended 28 unit limit for men and 21 for women, alcohol definitely undermines bone strength. A unit is half a pint of beer, a pub single of spirits or a small glass of wine.

Caffeine

Caffeine in excess – more than 6 cups of coffee a day – also damages bone, but is less harmful if taken as tea.

Medicines and other drugs

The safe rule is to avoid recreational drugs whose effect on bone is largely unknown, and any regular intake of over-the-counter drugs. You cannot always avoid the medicines your doctor prescribes for the benefit of your health, but at least if you are aware of the possible dangers you will not be pushing to increase the dose.

- Steroids are a boon in many disorders, but seriously damaging to your bones, reducing BMD, bone mass and the number of osteoblasts, the helpful bone-cells.
- Thyroxine, the chief thyroid hormone, often given in excess for underactive thyroid, speeds up bone turnover, increasing its loss.
- Anti-epileptics.
- Heparin, given to prevent clotting.
- Lithium, used in some serious psychiatric illness.
- Cytotoxics, used in chemotherapy for cancer.
- Phenothiazines, major tranquillizers used in schizophrenia.
- Tamoxifen, an anti-oestrogen, especially if given before the menopause.
- Theophylline, a life-saver in asthma.
- Nitrites, given for angina.
- Aluminium, present in some indigestion medicines.
- Iron overload.

If you are pregnant or breastfeeding, your bones are intimately involved in providing supplies of calcium for the newcomer's teeth and skeleton. Yours need consideration, too. Of course you will not be smoking or drinking alcohol, for your baby's sake. You will also have pepped up your diet (see p. 105) and will be doing exercises for the sake of your figure – all of this will benefit your bones.

Exercise

If you are into the menopause, have been ill, have tried serious slimming or have missed your periods at some stage in the past, your bone strength may be under par, and you cannot plunge into all the exercises suitable for a youngster. Similarly, if you know that you already have osteoporosis or you have had a fracture you must not take up a violent sport, but appropriate exercise is a bone-saver. The benefits include:

- slowing down the normal bone loss as you get older;
- the chance of increasing your bone mass – a little;
- improved physical well-being;
- increased self-confidence as you feel stronger;
- reduction in chronic back pain;
- less pain in the soft tissues – muscles, ligaments and tendons;
- less muscle fatigue, especially in your back;
- greater stability in standing and walking;

- better posture and balance;
- possibility of increased activity.

A recent study of people who had already had one fracture or phase of acute back pain compared the outcome in those who exercised systematically and those who did not bother. Only 3 of the exercise group had further vertebral fractures, compared with 10 of the non-exercisers; 13 exercisers had other types of fracture, compared with 16 non-exercisers. On the other hand, 32 exercisers lost most of their back pain, compared with 11 of the others.

After an acute phase of back pain or a fracture

Isometric exercises make a safe start – however soon. They comprise tensing your muscles but with no movement involved. Tighten each muscle or group of muscles in turn, holding the tension for a count of five. Repeat, say, ten times.

These exercises can do no harm, and they strengthen your muscles, making you less liable to have a fall, and secondarily benefit your bones. From these you can progress to exercises suggested by the physiotherapist or the doctor.

Don't:

- jog, jump or jolt your back or joints;
- twist your torso;
- lift anything heavy, or from low down;
- do flexion exercises, bending forwards, for instance to touch your toes;
- try to follow commercial exercise videos, unless they are specifically for patients with osteoporosis;
- use a rowing machine.

Walking is the kingpin of exercise that will benefit your bones. Use a Zimmer frame or walking sticks to get going, if necessary. Then move on.

Prescription for walking

First week	15 minutes a day
Second week	20 minutes a day
Third week	25 minutes a day

Then increase each week by five minutes a day until you reach one hour. Aim to continue with an hour's walk five times a week, indefinitely. Make sure your shoes are comfortable and of good quality.

Seniors

Your back, bottom and leg muscles tend to lose their strength with age. Exercise will prevent or correct this, and muscle tone, coordination, general agility and balance will also improve. If you are in your eighties or nineties, a set of exercises tailored to your individual needs will provide the maximum benefit: you need advice from a physiotherapist.

General purpose exercise programme

Assessment of your heart and lungs is a wise preliminary.

- *Walking*: swing your arms and walk a little faster than is comfortable.
- *Swimming*: any stroke is beneficial for your back muscles, but do not try breast stroke if you have had a hip fracture. Side stroke is the easiest in that case.
- *Cycling*: if you are using a stationary bicycle, pedal both forwards and backwards to use different muscles.

Neither swimming, cycling nor the use of some apparatus in a gym will benefit your bone strength directly since your body weight is supported, so do not let these be your main activities.

Specific back exercises

1 Elbows bent, at the side of your chest, pull your shoulder blades back. Hold for a count of five.
2 Hands behind the back of your head, pull your elbows backwards, breathe in deeply, hold and count to five. Relax.
3 Lie front down with a pillow under your chest and abdomen, arms by your sides. Lift your head and shoulders. Count five.
4 Kneel on hands and knees. Lift one leg at a time, holding it out straight, while you count five.
5 Lie on your back, and lift your legs, with your knees straight, one at a time and together, a few inches from the floor. Hold.
6 Lie flat on your back with your arms stretched above your head. Try to make yourself as long as possible, toes pointed and tummy pulled in. Hold.
7 Lie on your side and lift a straight leg sideways, to a count of five. Do the same on the other side.

You can expect a noticeable benefit within 6 to 12 weeks of daily exercises, or a little longer if you are hampered by arthritis or scoliosis (sideways curvature of the spine). After this intensive period of exercise, you can maintain your improvement with two or three sessions a week.

Adele

Adele was 59. She eked out the three sessions a week that she taught at the primary school with private piano pupils. It was a sedentary occupation and she had very little travelling to do. She had enjoyed team games as a child – netball, rounders – but now, apart from swimming on her holidays, she took hardly any exercise.

It had been since the change that she had noticed the backache, especially when she was leaning forwards over the piano, teaching. It became so bad that she went to the doctor. She diagnosed osteoporosis. Adele was already on HRT and ate what she regarded as an excellent diet. It provided plenty of calcium, but following her doctor's advice she cut down on red meat and substituted fish and cheese.

Her back continued to be painful until she chanced to have a chat with the PT teacher at the school, an anti-osteoporosis fanatic. She convinced Adele that the key to her problem was exercise and showed her some back-strengthening exercises. She also encouraged her through the effort and boredom of walking for 15 minutes every day, working up to 40 minutes three times a week. To her surprise Adele realized one day that she no longer had the troublesome pain. This was about six months later, but she cannot – ever – give up exercising or relapse is a certainty. However, she looks and feels better all round.

14

Prevention 2: Nourishing your bones

How can you make your bones strong and healthy, and ward off osteoporosis – or if it has already sneaked up on you, how can you keep it under control? The DIY answer is by your diet.

Our food is divided into two categories: *macronutrients* and *micronutrients*. Macronutrients comprise the three main classes: carbohydrates, the energy-suppliers like bread, rice and potatoes; proteins such as meat and cheese, essential for tissue-building and repair; and fats, such as cream and olive oil, which make a storage facility for extra fuel, and provide padding over the bony parts. You need substantial quantities of these foods, especially carbohydrates, to run your body.

By contrast you require only tiny amounts of the micronutrients – micro is Greek for small – but your life and health depend on them. They are the vitamins and minerals. Your bones need several of each, but the two crucial ingredients are calcium and vitamin D, and all bone-saving diets depend on these two. They work together.

Calcium

When the human species evolved, in equatorial East Africa, there was a superabundance of both calcium and vitamin D. The diet of primitive man was based on hunting and gathering berries, nuts and roots, and later it included herding animals and drinking their milk. It provided 2000 to 4000 mg of calcium daily, compared with a measly average of 500 mg in today's Western diet. To avoid overload, the intestine was geared to absorb only about 5 per cent of the intake, and this is the situation still. When farming came in, roughly 10,000 years ago, it meant that people began relying on cereal crops for their nourishment. They grew – and we still grow – those that provide the most carbohydrate, regardless of their micronutrient content. They contain very little calcium, and even the fruit and vegetables we cultivate today are favoured for the sugar and starch they provide.

Our farming ancestors of thousands of years ago – probably the women – realized something was lacking in their diet. The Central American Indians took to adding lime to their corn meal and those in the Andes used powdered rock to pep up their cereal gruel. In the Second World War we did the same sort of thing in the UK. We added calcium carbonate (chalk) to the wheat flour to make the National Loaf.

Pregnant women in the more remote areas of South-East Asia still drink a calcium-rich liquid made from soaking bones in vinegar. We are not so very advanced after all, with our calcium supplements, which are particularly necessary during pregnancy and breastfeeding. In addition, the body has tricks of its own to preserve mothers' bones. It absorbs more of the available calcium and excretes less. Unfortunately there is no similar leg-up to help older people and their bones.

How much calcium you need – daily doses (US recommendations)

Children aged 1–5 years	800 mg
Children from 6 years	800–1200 mg
Girls aged 9–20	900–1200 mg
Boys aged 12–22	900–1200 mg
Teenagers to age 24	1200–1500 mg
Pregnant and breastfeeding women	1200–1500 mg
if also a teenager	1500 mg
Women aged 24–45	1000 mg
Men aged 24–65	1000 mg
Women over 45 on HRT	1000 mg
Women over 45 not on HRT	1500 mg
Men and women over 65	1500 mg

What happens to the calcium we eat or drink?

A small proportion is absorbed. It is vital for your bones that this is enough to meet their needs.

- Adults manage to retain 4–8 per cent of their intake.
- Teenagers and young adults retain 20 per cent.
- Pregnant and nursing mothers also retain 20 per cent.
- Infants retain 40 per cent.

If supplies are inadequate during the growth period the bones are much the same size but the cortex is thin and the honeycomb of the trabecular bone is scanty – with a future risk of fractures. Between the ages of 18 and 50 there is a positive link between the amount of calcium you take in and your bone mass.

From 50 onwards your intestines absorb less calcium and the bone mass – the total amount of bone in your body – gradually diminishes, however much of the mineral you swallow. There is an individual threshold above which no extra calcium can be absorbed, but it is only with intakes of over 2000 mg a day that side-effects may occur. Constipation and occasionally other disturbances of the digestive system are then possible.

You can only store calcium in your bones, so they are dependent on a constant supply from outside to make up for the natural losses. Calcium is lost:

- in the urine;
- in sweat;
- in skin, nails and hair.

What improves the absorption of calcium

- Eating carbohydrates at the same time as the calcium-containing food, for instance bread and cheese.
- An illness called sarcoidosis.
- Oestrogen, for instance in hormone replacement therapy (HRT).
- Exercise helps the calcium get into the bones, but it does not counteract a low intake of calcium or any of the factors which inhibit its absorption. Too much exercise is counterproductive.

What hinders the absorption of calcium

- Growing older, especially past 50.
- Lack of sex hormone, for instance with the menopause or after some gynaecological operations, or in the case of men, a shortage of testosterone.
- Some chronic illnesses: Crohn's disease, coeliac disease, kidney disease.

Medicines which interfere with the absorption of calcium

- Tetracyclines, for instance Achromycin.
- Anti-epileptics, for example phenobarbitone.
- Corticosteroids, for instance prednisolone.
- Aluminium in indigestion mixtures.
- Thyroxine.

Medicines increasing the loss of calcium in the urine

All those hindering absorption, plus:
- 'loop' water tablets, such as frusemide;
- isoniazid, used in the treatment of tuberculosis.

Dangers and disadvantages that can crop up in your diet

- Excess of animal protein: this speeds up bone turnover and increases the loss of calcium in the urine. Vegetarians need less calcium than meat-eaters.
- Excess of phosphates, which compete with calcium. They are found in fast foods, processed foods with additives and cola drinks.
- Caffeine, especially plentiful in filter coffee but also in instant, tea, chocolate drinks. Tea is less harmful because it boosts oestrogen; carob can substitute for chocolate flavour; and milk in your coffee can make up for the reduced absorption of calcium.

- Oxalates: green vegetables can be a good source if they do not contain oxalates which bind the calcium so that it cannot be absorbed. Oxalates are present in spinach, asparagus, parsley, sorrel, strawberries, dandelion leaves and rhubarb.
- Phytates prevent the absorption of calcium in a similar way to oxalates. They are found in the outer husks of cereal grain, importantly wheat and especially, oatmeal. Not all Scots run short of calcium, probably because some are more liberal with the milk on their porridge, and rye contains an enzyme called phytase, which splits up the phytates. White bread, in which the outer part of the grain is milled off, provides more calcium than brown or wholemeal. Phytates also inhibit the absorption of iron, magnesium, boron and zinc which are needed in minute – trace – amounts for healthy bones.
- Sodium, in the form of salt, increases the loss of calcium in the urine. It is found in soy and other sauces and pickles, ham, bacon, salt fish, anchovies, Marmite, Bovril – and cornflakes. A sprinkle of Parmesan cheese substitutes for salt – and adds calcium to the dish.
- Alcohol in excess prevents the utilization of calcium because of its effect on the liver. Often this is made worse by the cigarettes which may accompany the drink.

Vitamin D (cholecalciferol)

Like calcium, vitamin D was available to early man in excess, but by a different route. Then, as now, we only obtained a little of our vitamin D from our food, but we can manufacture it in our skin by a photochemical reaction using the ultra-violet rays of the sun. In the part of Africa where the great human adventure began, there was sunlight galore and the main danger was of the toxic effect of too much of the vitamin. This can be fatal, with symptoms like meningitis. Dark skin evolved to screen out some of the potentially harmful UV rays.

The people who went to live in the more temperate climate of the northern latitudes, on the other hand, developed paler skins so that they could get as much of the ultra-violet effect as possible. The sunshine is less intense farther from the equator. The rays are more horizontal, and have to pass through more of earth's atmosphere, including its pollution, before reaching anyone's skin – with a loss of ultra-violet en route.

Another factor is the colder northern climate. Like our forebears, we cover most of our skin with clothing, preventing the sun's rays falling on it – particularly when we are elderly and frail. Again, older people tend to spend much of their time indoors, especially in retirement homes, shielded even more from ultra-violet rays which are filtered out by glass windows.

Yet it is the seniors who need the sunlight most, since their skins are less efficient at manufacturing the vitamin.

It is noteworthy that more hip fractures occur in the sunless midwinter months than in summer, and they are more prevalent in the north of Scotland than on the sunnier south coast.

While our bodies are designed by nature to protect us from too much vitamin D and calcium, we in the West are at risk of getting too little of either, and by 60-plus we are certain to be running short. The use of sunscreens past the age of 45 to 50 can leave you deprived of vitamin D, and older people should never use them, except on a Mediterranean holiday.

Sharon

Sharon, at 32, was literally moonlighting – working in a private hospital at night and for the NHS by day. She managed to sneak enough sleep (nearly) in the quiet periods at night, but she was seldom able to get outdoors. She was concerned to keep her figure, already very slim, and filled herself up with vast quantities of fizzy cola drinks, a sure-fire way of cutting down on calcium. She would not dream of having milk in any form. She was saving for a holiday in Switzerland.

Skiing holidays are notorious for broken bones, but Sharon's wrist and ankle fractures followed a very mild tumble. She had osteoporosis – brought on by lack of ultra-violet light on her skin and lack of calcium from her diet. The breaks healed quickly but it will take many months to restore the strength to her bones.

Prescription for sunlight

Sixty, 30, or even just 15 minutes daily of exposure of the face, neck and forearms to sunlight is probably enough for a 70-year-old's need for vitamin D. The amount produced is around a third of what it would have been at age 20. You can burn your skin, but you cannot cause vitamin D toxicity from sunlight alone. It can only occur with excessive use of vitamin tablets or fish liver oil.

Ultra-violet rays do not produce instant cholecalciferol, but set off a process which takes three or four days, longer in older people. The vitamin is stored in the liver, which must be healthy if it is to play its part.

Vitamin D in your food

Although the main source of cholecalciferol is your private factory in the skin, you can get a certain amount in your diet. As far back as the eighteenth century, cod liver oil was established as a folk remedy for weak bones. Its value as a nourishing food for old and young was highlighted by

Professor Hughes Bennett in Edinburgh a century later, and Trousseau in France used it in children with rickets. However it was not until 1931 that preparations of the pure vitamin were made – simultaneously in England and Germany. It was only then that the amount in various foods could be measured.

League table for vitamin D

Fish liver oil (in micrograms per 100 grams)

Swordfish liver oil	25,000 (first catch your swordfish)
Halibut liver oil	500–10,000
Cod liver oil	200–750
Shark liver oil	30–125

Ordinary foods

Fish: herrings, salmon, pilchards and sardines	5–45
Eggs	1.25
Yolks only	4–10
Vitaminized spread	2–9
Cheese	0.3
Milk	0.1
Olive oil	nil
Cereals, vegetables and fruit	nil
Meat and white fish	negligible

A certain amount of fat is necessary for the absorption of vitamin D. It is processed in the liver, and the final residue disposed of in the motions. Its essential job is to promote the absorption of calcium and phosphorus. Calcium phosphate is the raw material used by the osteoblasts to build and restore bone tissue.

Other important micronutrients

Vitamin K

Some elderly victims of fractured hip turn out to be short of this vitamin. It is used in the manufacture of bone proteins and for normal clotting of the blood. It is found in dark green vegetables such as kale, spinach, alfalfa – and also cauliflower. There is none in meat or dairy products.

Vitamin C

This is needed for the production of collagen, the fibrous background tissue of bone and skin. A lack of it causes scurvy – and osteoporosis. You can find it in citrus fruits, soft fruits, pineapple, tomatoes and salad vegetables and best of all in blackcurrants, in any form.

Bantu

The Bantu men of South Africa do not bother eating fruit and vegetables but concentrate on ale made in huge iron pots. By middle age many of them suffer from siderosis (iron overload), scurvy, alcoholism – and osteoporosis.

B vitamins: B6, pyridoxine and B12, cobalamin

Vitamin B6 works in conjunction with vitamin C to make collagen. You get it from meat, wheat bran and Marmite.

B12 is vital to the metabolism of every cell in your body, and especially where re-building is going on. It is available in all animal foods but in none of the vegetable type. Vegans can become seriously ill, but intractable backache is the likeliest result.

Checklist for calcium in your food

Dairy products are the key to your calcium supply, but if you are unlucky enough to be short of lactase, the enzyme needed to digest milk sugar, you must find other sources. The same applies if you cut down your milk intake severely as an adult, either because you dislike it or you are watching your weight. The list below shows the calcium content of a wide range of common foods.

Dairy products

Milk (150 ml / $\frac{1}{4}$ pint):

Full cream	180 mg (98 calories)
Skimmed, including dried	195 mg (50 calories)
Longlife	180 mg (98 calories)
Evaporated	420 mg (237 calories)
Condensed skimmed	570 mg (400 calories)
Goats'	100 mg (100 calories)

Amounts per 100 g / $3\frac{1}{2}$ oz:

Yogurt, natural	180 mg (52 calories)
Yogurt, low fat, flavoured with fruit	170 mg (40 calories)
Egg custard	130 mg (118 calories)
Dairy ice cream	130 mg (150 calories)
Cream, single	79 mg (212 calories)
Cream, double	50 mg (447 calories)

Cheese (50 g / 2 oz):

Cheddar	400 mg (203 calories)
Edam	370 mg (152 calories)
Feta	360 mg (122 calories)
Stilton	180 mg (230 calories)
Danish blue	290 mg (177 calories)
Processed	350 mg (155 calories)
Cream cheese	49 mg (219 calories)
Cottage	60 mg (96 calories)
Parmesan (25 g / 1 oz grated)	305 mg (102 calories)
Milk chocolate bar (56 g / 2 oz)	123 mg (250 calories)
Mars bar	90 mg (293 calories)

Vegetables

Amounts per 112 g / 4 oz, cooked:

Spinach	179 mg
Parsley	200 mg
Asparagus	13 mg
Beetroot	40 mg

(Very little of the calcium from these 4 is available because of oxalates.)

Curly kale	150 mg
Okra	220 mg
Spring greens	84 mg
Cabbage	43 mg
Baked beans	59 mg
Spring onions, raw (50 g / 2 oz)	70 mg

Potatoes and most other plant foods either contain very little calcium or it is unavailable because of oxalates or phytates.

Nuts and seeds

Amounts per 100 g / $3\frac{1}{2}$ oz:

Almonds	250 mg
Brazil nuts	180 mg
Walnuts	60 mg
Hazelnuts	140 mg
Peanuts	61 mg
Chestnuts	46 mg
Coconut (fresh)	13 mg
Sesame seeds	670 mg

Fish

Amounts per 100 g / $3\frac{1}{2}$ oz:

Whitebait, fried (56 g / 2 oz)	482 mg
Haddock, fried	110 mg
Cod, cooked	80 mg
Plaice, cooked	93 mg
Salmon, canned	195 mg
Sardines, canned	460 mg
Pilchards, canned	168 mg
Tuna, canned	7 mg
Prawns, cooked	110 mg
Oysters, raw	190 mg

Meat

Amounts per 100 g / $3\frac{1}{2}$ oz:

Steak pudding	110 mg
Moussaka	88 mg
Beef sausage, grilled	73 mg

(Chicken, turkey, duck, beef, lamb, ham – amounts too small to be useful)

Egg, one	26 mg
Egg, scrambled with milk	30 mg

Bread and cakes

Amounts per 100 g / $3\frac{1}{2}$ oz:

Bread	
Wholemeal	23 mg
White	100 mg
Malt	94 mg
Scones (made with baking powder)	620 mg
Gingerbread	210 mg
Victoria sponge	140 mg
Fruit cake	60 mg
Bun	90 mg
Chocolate biscuits	110 mg
Semi-sweet and water biscuits	120 mg
Shortbread	97 mg

Fruit

Amounts per 100 g / 3½ oz:

Orange, one, according to size	40–60 mg
Raspberries	40 mg
Strawberries (contain oxalates)	22 mg
Blackberries	63 mg
Dried raisins	61 mg
Dried figs	280 mg

Sugar, honey and syrup

Only molasses and black treacle contain appreciable calcium.

Molasses (25 g / 1 oz)	171 mg
Black treacle	125 mg

Oils, fats and spreads

Only butter contains more than a trace of calcium.

Butter (100 g / 3½ oz)	25 mg

Drinks

Only milk-based drinks and strong ale contain an appreciable amount.

Strong ale 300 ml (½ pint)	42 mg

Alternative therapy recommendations for osteoporosis

- Nettle
- Slippery elm
- Horsetail
- Alfalfa
- Burdock
- Sage
- Borage
- Evening primrose
- Blackcurrant
- Ginseng
- Soya
- Green vegetable and carrot juice

There is no scientific evidence to show that any of the herbal remedies named has an effect on osteoporosis or the risk of it, but you could be one of the lucky ones who feels markedly better taking a particular plant remedy. They are unlikely to do you any harm, so why not give them a try if you are so inclined.

Minerals

Copper, selenium, manganese, magnesium, boron, silicon. There is no reason to think that the necessary traces of these substances are not easily provided by an ordinary diet, vegetarian or other, but they may be bought in health food shops in tablet form.

Useful addresses

United Kingdom

National Osteoporosis Society
Camerton
Bath BA2 0PJ
Tel: 01761 471771
Fax: 01761 471104
Helpline: 0845 4500 230
Email: *info@nos.org.uk*
www.nos.org.uk

Age Concern England
1268 London Road
London SW16 4ER
Tel: 020-8765 7200
Helpline: 0800 00 99 66
www.ageconcern.org.uk

Republic of Ireland

Irish Osteoporosis Society (IOS)
33 Pearse Street
Dublin 2
Ireland
Tel: 00 353 1 677 4267
Email: *info@irishosteoporosis.ie*
www.irishosteoporosis.ie

USA

National Osteoporosis Foundation
1232 22nd Street N.W.
Washington
DC 20037–1292
Tel: (202) 223-2226
Email: *subgroup@nof.org* for support groups
www.nof.org

National Institute of Health Osteoporosis and Related Bone Diseases
National Resource Center
2 AMS Circle
Bethesda
MD 20892–3679
Tel: (202) 223-0344
Toll-free: 800-624-BONE
Fax: (202) 293-2356
TTY: (202) 466-4315
Email: *NIAMSBONEINFO@mail.nih.gov*
www.osteo.org

Australia

Osteoporosis Australia
Level 1
52 Parramatta Road
Forest Lodge
NSW 2037
GPO Box 121, Sydney NSW 2001
Tel: (02) 9518 8140
Fax: (02) 9518 6306
www.osteoporosis.org.au

Osteoporosis New South Wales
13 Harold Street
North Parramatta
NSW 2151
Tel: (02) 9683 1622
Fax: (02) 9683 1633
Toll-free: 1800 242 141
www.osteoporosis.org.au

There are also branches for Queensland, Western Australia, and South Australia.

New Zealand

Osteoporosis New Zealand
PO Box 688
Wellington
New Zealand
Tel: (04) 499 4862
Fax: (04) 499 4863
www.bones.org.nz

Canada

Osteoporosis Canada
1090 Don Mills Road, Suite 301
Toronto
Ontario
M36 3R6
Tel: (416) 696-2663
Fax: (416) 696-2673
Toll-free (English): 1-800-463-6842
Use this number to find the self-help group closest to you.
Toll-free (French): 1-800-977-1778
Email: *info@osteoporosis.ca*
www.osteoporosis.ca

Chapters (branches) in: Alberta, Calgary, Fredericton, Manitoba, Winnipeg, Peel, Peterborough, Quebec and Saskatchewan.

Index

activation 4
Adele 103–4
adjustment disorder 96
adolescence 35, 59, 62
Africa 36
alcohol 23, 26, 30, 38, 44, 92, 100
alendronate 68, 70, 73
Alex 44–5
algodystrophy 85
alternative therapy 114
Andrew 16
androgens 27
Angela 20–1
anorexia 2
  nervosa 24, 44, 53, 77
antacids 38
anticonvulsants 31, 38, 49
antidepressants 95
anti-sex hormone drugs 31–2
anxiety 93–4
arthritis 40, 80, 89, 91
Astrid 8–9
astronauts 98

backache 9, 42
balance 4
Bantu 13, 36
Ben 96
Beryl 95
BGP: bone Gla protein 49, 56
bloating 65
BMD: bone mineral density 9, 19, 25, 29, 42, 47, 54, 71
bran 6, 38
bread 113

breast-feeding 25–6, 62
Bryony 29

caffeine 38, 100, 107
cake 113
calcitonin 23, 29, 55–8
calcium 5, 6, 22, 23, 25, 27, 29, 40, 55, 59, 62, 105
causalgia 21
chemotherapy 38, 44, 101
Chinese 36
cholecalciferol 7, 108
cigarettes *see* tobacco
Claire 55
coeliac disease 6, 33, 107
coffee 30, 107
cognitive therapy 95
collapse 19
constipation 12, 65
cooking 83
cortex 3
counselling 95
coupling 4
Crohn's disease 33–4, 107
Cushing, Harvey 28
cycling 103

density *see* BMD
depression 12, 40, 84, 90, 95
DEXA test 39, 44, 46, 49
diabetes 18, 26, 33, 44, 51, 64
'dowager's hump' 12, 22, 45
drinks 114
driving 83

DVT: deep vein thrombosis 80, 87

Edna 96–7
eggs 113
endometriosis 51
Erica 52
etidronate 30, 54, 68, 70, 73
Evelyn 12–13
exercise 7, 16, 24, 40, 44, 81–2, 98–9
  isometric 102

falls 27, 30, 32, 75, 76, 88
fatigue 15
  tissue 5
fear 12
fluoride 59–60
food 6–7
formation 4, 32
fracture
  ankle 86
  backbone 87
  Colles' 16–17, 88
  crush 1, 8, 10, 19, 57, 60
  endplate 10
  hip 1, 8, 13–16, 53, 75
  incident 10
  prevalence 10
  metatarsal 86
  shin-bone 86
  shoulder 17, 86
  vertebral 8, 9–10, 16, 19, 26
  wedge 10, 12, 27
  wrist 19, 20–1 (*see also* Colles')
fruit 114
frusemide 107

gallstones 51
Geoffrey 23
George 27
glucocorticoids 28
growth hormone 59

haemophilia 34
headaches 51
height 10, 11
Helen 57
heparin 31, 44, 101
hemiarthroplasty 17, 79, 81, 85
hiatus hernia 12
hip protector 9, 40
hip replacement 9, 15, 80, 85
HRT: hormone replacement therapy 27, 38, 47, 50–3, 95
hydroxyapatite 65
hydroxyproline 4, 49, 56
hypercalcaemia 64
hypogonadism 26, 54
hypothyroidism 31
hysterectomy 38, 47

ibuprofen 58
ileus 11
internal fixation 80

jaws 19
Joan 97

kidney
  disease 33, 44, 54, 107
  stones 54
Kirsty 65
kyphosis 12, 22

leukaemia 32, 34
lithium 32, 101
Luke 33
lung cancer 34
lymphoma 34

Maggie 80
magnesium 60
Malays 36
Malcolm 77
mammogram 55
Maoris 13, 36

mass, bone 5, 19, 25, 42, 45, 47, 62
matrix 3, 4
meat 113
medroxyprogesterone 58–9
memory 40
menopause 5, 6, 19, 20, 42, 44
methotrexate 32
Michael 84
Midge 100
mineralization 4
minerals 114
Miriam 94
morphometry 46
multiple sclerosis 2, 33, 44

nandrolone 54, 59
Naomi 39
National Loaf 105
NSAIDs: non-steroidal anti-inflammatory drugs 11, 33, 58, 81
numbness 11
nuts and seeds 112

oestrogen 18, 20, 24, 38, 50, 58
oophorectomy 56
osteoblasts 3, 20, 22, 29, 30
osteocalcin 49
osteoclasts 3, 4, 20, 29, 32
osteocytes 3
osteogenesis imperfecta 9, 34, 68
osteomalacia 7, 9, 31
osteopenia 7, 35, 44, 58
oxalates 38, 108, 112

Paget's disease 33, 49, 56, 67
pamidronate 70
Parkinson's disease 34, 40, 90
periods 44, 52
phosphates 107
phytates 6, 108
polymyalgia rheumatica 29

prednisolone 29, 107
pregnancy 25–6, 51
progesterone 58
prosthesis 79
protein 105, 107
psychotherapy 95
puberty 36, 54

QCT: quantitative computerized tomography 47
QSM: quantitative spinal morphometry 46
QUS: quantitative ultrasound 47, 49

race 36
radiogrammetry 45–6
radiotherapy 38, 44
raloxifene 54
reduction 17
resorption 4, 6, 19, 31, 33, 48, 68
reversal 4
rheumatoid arthritis 2, 21, 28, 33, 69
rhubarb 38
rickets 7, 9
risedronate 73
Rita 17

salcatonin 57
salt 29, 108
Samson 60
screening 42
Sharon 109
Singh Index 46
SERM: selective (o)estrogen receptor modulator 54
slimming 24, 62
smoking *see* tobacco
sodium 38, 108
SSRI: selective serotonin re-uptake inhibitor 95

stanozolol 59
sterilization 38
steroids 28, 38, 44, 64, 77, 101
   anabolic 59
strontium ranelate 73–4
sunlight, sunshine 16, 36, 40,
   109
sunscreens 109
Svetlana 24
Sweden 36
swimming 103
Sylvia 89

tamoxifen 31, 58, 101
teriparatide 73
Tessa 46
testosterone 27, 29, 53–4, 59
   implant 45
tetracycline 38, 64, 107
theophylline 101
thiazide diuretics 60
Third Age 63
thyrotoxicosis 33, 48
thyroxine 31, 38, 101
tobacco 16, 23, 26, 30–1, 38, 45,
   92, 100
trabeculum, trabecular 3, 8, 19,
   21

tranquillizers 31–2
twins 25

ultrasound 43, 56
   quantitative 47, 49

vegetables 112
vegetarians 107
vertebral fractures *see* fractures
vitamins
   B group 111
   C 38, 110
   D 6–7, 20, 22, 25, 27, 32, 38,
     60, 108, 109–10
   K 38, 110

walking 103
Ward's triangle 46
wheat 6
   bran 6, 38
wholemeal 6, 38, 113
Winifred 72
wrist 16–17, 21, 27

X-ray 8, 11, 16, 17, 45

Zimmer 82, 102
zinc 38, 108